THE BALANCE CONCEPT IN HEALTH AND NURSING

A UNIVERSAL APPROACH TO CARE AND SURVIVAL

Daisy Magalit Rodriguez

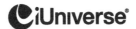

THE BALANCE CONCEPT IN HEALTH AND NURSING
A UNIVERSAL APPROACH TO CARE AND SURVIVAL

iUniverse books may be ordered through booksellers or by contacting:

iUniverse
1663 Liberty Drive
Bloomington, IN 47403
www.iuniverse.com
1-800-Authors (1-800-288-4677)

Because of the dynamic nature of the Internet, any web addresses or links contained in this book may have changed since publication and may no longer be valid. The views expressed in this work are solely those of the author and do not necessarily reflect the views of the publisher, and the publisher hereby disclaims any responsibility for them.

Any people depicted in stock imagery provided by Thinkstock are models, and such images are being used for illustrative purposes only.
Certain stock imagery © Thinkstock.

ISBN: 978-1-4917-2222-0 (sc)
ISBN: 978-1-4917-2223-7 (e)

Library of Congress Control Number: 2014901891

Print information available on the last page.

iUniverse rev. date: 07/29/2015

DEDICATION

To the most important people in my life—my husband, Ruben; my two children, Robyn and Reuben, and my three precious grandsons, Amado, Aiden and Eli. You have been my inspiration and give me balance as I travel down the pathway of life. You are the reasons for this book.

-Daisy Magalit Rodriguez, MN, MPA, RN

EPIGRAPH: A POEM

TO FLORENCE

In the glow of your lamp
you walk among the wounded
wiping sweat from feverish brows,
whispering words of comfort,
holding a limp hand.

You turn to acknowledge
a greeting, a smile, a nod;
utter a silent prayer for a dying man
breathing his last.

Distant gunfires barely drown
the words of someone's plea:
"Please tell my wife I love her,
all my life I hold her dear".

You nod your head in silence
knowing words would not suffice;
wondering if he will ever see
tomorrow's light of day.

Pain and suffering you see everywhere
still you hurry your feet to reach
the last soldier moaning,
to stem blood from gaping wounds.

The roars of cannons draw near,
It's the enemy sure to kill.
But duty calls, you persevere
for friend or foe you care.

In the glow of your lamp
you cast a long shadow,
for all those who will follow
like a beacon for tomorrow.

Your words echo through the years
never fading, always reminding,
that we have a solemn duty
to those in our keeping.

Florence, your name is on our lips,
your beauty is in your soul;
Your deeds always remembered
even in our slumber.

Your pledge is one we shall
in our hearts forever keep;
not forgetting, always remembering
as long as the nightingale sings.

A poem by Daisy Magalit Rodriguez (2004)

ACKNOWLEDGMENTS

This book could not have been written if not for the numerous people throughout my life who have guided me, mentored me, appreciated me, gave me support when I was faltering with self-doubt, comforted me when I was sad, and loved me unconditionally despite my human imperfections. They are the people who have given me balance in my life and provided me with the courage to seek what lay beyond the mountain of challenges people encounter in their daily lives.

First, my family, especially my husband Ruben, who has endured hours without my company while I was busy at my computer trying to put elusive ideas into words. To my children, Robyn and Reuben, you grew up into remarkable adults while your dad and I were trying to make better lives for us after immigrating to this country we now call home. You are not only amazing individuals but also gave us three beautiful grandchildren. Thank you too, Val. Robyn, your drive to achieve academic excellence has inspired me to fulfill a long-time dream of writing a book, following your footsteps. To my sister Cheerie, my gratitude for being there for me and sharing your love of nature. To my older brothers and sisters, you have been my compass through those years when we were growing up. I would not be what I am without the strength of our bond and our love for each other.

To the numerous nurses I have known throughout my nursing career, each one of whom have touched my life in many ways, I am grateful to have been part of yours. To the nurses who work in the trenches day in and day out saving lives, caring for sick patients, and supporting families—you are the real heroes. You deserve my respect and admiration. There are also several who stand out in my long list of nursing colleagues: Professor Judy Berg of the University of Arizona, my co-author and co-investigator in two research projects, my utmost gratitude for your scholarly review of my book and writing the foreword; Dr. Kathy Abriam Yago of San Jose State University, thank you always for your support; Carolina De Guzman, my mentor, long-time friend, collaborator in our research and writing projects, organizational leader, and role-model, I cannot thank you enough for your support and friendship thru the years. To my colleagues at Unitek College, I derived some insights into the development of my ideas through your passion for teaching and nursing. You have inspired ideas that contributed in many ways to this book.

The diagrams I developed were important illustrations of my concepts. Tom Santos, graphic designer extraordinaire, made those models exactly to my specifications. In my opinion, nobody could have done a better job. You told me that you just want me to be successful. It was wonderful to hear that from anyone—thanks so much.

Balance, applied to all areas of my life, has given me a sense of purpose. It is elusive and sometimes fleeting. But fragile as it may seem, it is the thread that connects us all as human beings. No man is an island, the author John Donne once wrote. To be able to shed some insight into this phenomena is reward enough for me. I hope this book will help, even in a small way, in developing that body of knowledge unique to nursing for the next generation.

Daisy Magalit Rodriguez, MN, MPA, RN

CONTENTS

LIST OF DIAGRAMS AND TABLES

FOREWORD

Balance is a universal concept with myriad meanings and interpretations. The author of this text perceives balance as an intangible concept, yet one that can be measured and described in terms of behavior or activity of the organism plus the structure or system in which it occurs. Equilibrium, harmony, symmetry, equality, and stability are sometimes used synonymously with the term balance, and yet these terms may be thought of as attributes rather than synonyms. Carefully thought out in relationship to health, balance is described in this text as having five essential elements: adaptation, equilibrium, homeostasis, health, and needs working synergistically to achieve survival. *These* elements were described individually in the first chapter *of Part 1.* The primary focus of the first part of the book is to understand the universality of balance, internal and external environments that have influence on the concept, and to describe balance and behavior, including balance-seeking behaviors, and finally how balance relates to culture.

In the second part of the book, the author made a strong case for balance being central to nursing. Indeed, much of this text is dedicated to discussions that place balance within *a* health-illness continuum and how this is related to nursing and its theoretical underpinnings. For example, nursing theorists, such as Florence Nightingale, Betty Neuman, Dorothy Johnson, Sister Callista Roy, Martha Rogers, Margaret Newman, Madeleine Leininger, and Jean Watson, embraced balance as an essential component of their explanations of health and illness with emphasis on environment, systems, behavior, adaptation, etc. A controversial critique of the nursing profession has been that it borrows theories from sociology, psychology, and other disciplines. Although some consider this a strength and basis for inter-professional collaboration, the addition of a nursing theory on balance affords a wider array of theories appropriate for use by researchers, educators, and clinicians within the profession. As well, this theory on balance can be utilized by other professions as a legitimate basis for their scientific endeavors.

Perhaps the greatest strength of the concept of balance is that it can serve as a framework for nursing practice. The entire discussion of the nursing process in a balance nursing model places nursing practice in that context. Core concepts in the model contribute to the ultimate goal of achieving the highest level of balance by utilizing the nursing process which begins with assessment leading to a nursing diagnosis, planning, applying appropriate interventions, then evaluating to determine intervention effectiveness at modifying behavior. Failure to achieve the desired outcomes requires reassessment and cycling through the process again.

All theories are evolutionary and unlikely to remain static. Instead, the revisions that result from testing and use serve to strengthen our understanding of the elements and their relationships. Follow-up to the proposed balance theoretical model is required to validate its elements. This can be achieved by utilizing it as the underpinning of nursing research, scholarship, and practice. It will be interesting to observe its evolution over time.

Judith A. Berg, PhD, RN, WHNP-BC, FAAN, FAANP
Clinical Professor
The University of Arizona College of Nursing
Tucson, Arizona

PREFACE

When I retired from my teaching job, I knew I wanted to do something more productive instead of just sitting on a rocking chair. There was one thing I had always wanted to do: write a book as part of my legacy to my children and grandchildren. But the question that required serious consideration was about what I should write.

I could write about my childhood, growing up in the small town of Numancia in the province of Aklan in the Philippines. Those were halcyon days of my youth, where I and my older siblings—two brothers and two sisters—spent our summers playing hide-and-seek on moonlight nights, wading in the clear brook near our house looking for snails, or with our neighbor friends, built make-shift playhouses out of banana leaves and coconut palms. No matter that we did not have shoes, except wooden clogs, or new outfits to wear to church. We were happy just being together sharing whatever we had, even a copy of an old magazine, and talking about going to distant places.

Our mother died when I was very young—a mere three years old, not even remembering her face except in my dreams. My eldest sister, just nine years older than myself, became my surrogate mother. We still have that kind of relationship to this day, even in our graying years. Our father was a municipal treasurer in town, a man known for his unflinching honesty, generosity, and devotion to his five young children. I don't know how our dad raised us on his meager salary but we did survive the post—World War II years. I remember sharing a small can of evaporated milk among the five of us—two teaspoons each, mixed with a cup of hot water for breakfast. Sugar was a luxury, only broiled dried fish and boiled vegetables. I often wondered if I had been smarter if I only had more nutritious food that nourished my brain.

Surviving a whole slew of childhood diseases was in itself, a struggle for survival. I and my older brother, two years older, were always the victims of these childhood diseases—chicken pox, mumps, measles, head lice, infections, etc. Of course, being the youngest, I had the privilege of eating saltine crackers and on occasion, a piece of Sunkist orange that my father sacrificed to take from our daily food allowance. By the grace of God, we all finished high school and college with top honors. After graduating as high school valedictorian, I passed a government exam by the Philippine National Science Development Board. I was awarded a full scholarship to go to the most prestigious school in the country—the University of the Philippines. Attending the university led me to a multitude of paths that took me half-way around the world and opened up a new world of opportunities. I ended up becoming a nurse and got to the land of my dreams—the United States of America. I married a charming husband and raised two great children—a daughter and a son. This is another story I would like to write someday. My daughter, now a university sociology professor, has published her second book and working on her third. I have three lovely grandsons. God has been good to me. I feel truly blest.

My professional nursing career led me to serve in top leadership capacities on both the local chapter and national organizations of Philippine nurses in the United States. As president of the Philippine Nurses Association of Northern California, Inc. and as a member of the Executive Board of the Philippine Nurses Association of America, I strove to give back what has been given to me with my knowledge, skills, and training. I found that service for the advancement of my professional nursing organizations and my community helped me find a sense of fulfillment and balance.

To me, the greatest gift for mankind is the gift of the tenacity of the human spirit, the innate will to survive against all odds. Where did this come from? In what repository of the brain is that spirit hidden? Why do we struggle to survive? What impulse always leads us to preserve ourselves and keep us striving for something better?

These were the questions that I pondered upon throughout my adult life but could not find any good explanation. Science offers some in the study of human behavior and the human body. But nothing comes even close to understanding the phenomena of the secrets to human survival. All I know to this day is about what I can speak from personal experience, my striving to make my life as balanced as possible and to do more than just merely survive. Life is full of possibilities to let it slide by without savoring the moment. I call this a striving for balance. This is a subject that I decided to embark upon and why I felt compelled to write this book.

The subject of balance in this book is not as much about balancing one's life but more about the theoretical concept of balance. I perceived that there must be forces present everywhere that maintain balance. The knowledge and experiences I have accumulated over my lifetime seem to find a locus in that one concept. I wondered, could this have anything to do with survival? As I delved deeper into the subject, I found more evidences that indeed, balance supports survival. One has to have the elements of balance to survive on earth: the physiological process of homeostasis to regulate and maintain our internal physiologic balance; the balancing influences of equilibrium to find the optimal level of stability, harmony, and well-being; the innate ability to adapt to environmental changes and surmount the harshness of nature; the gratification of needs from the basic physiologic to man's highest aspirations;

and the preservation of health that is tantamount to life preservation. All these combined, provide some rational and plausible explanation for why humans like you and I have continued to survive and will continue to survive far into the future. And yet, it still does not fully explain that spark in the human spirit that pushes humans to be more than the sum of their individual parts.

My background as a nurse and an educator was instrumental in my pursuit of devising a theoretical model that would be useful in my profession and to those who will come after me. In school, I learned about the works of Florence Nightingale, the pioneering nurse in England who set a different course for the profession. Her innovative thinking became the foundation of modern nursing. Nearly a decade ago, I wrote a poem dedicated to her. Such has been my admiration for a nurse who called her profession a "calling". Many others in the history of nursing have responded to this call and left their footprints for future nurses to follow.

When I started writing this book on balance, I knew intuitively that there was a connection to nursing. However, I did not quite know how I could connect all the concepts related to balance and bring nursing into the picture. I found the key in the concept of health—health as one of the core elements of balance, an ingredient if you will, of the recipe for survival. The connection became crystal clear to me with the realization that nursing practices within a health-illness continuum and provides the interventions that could preserve life, protect life and maintain life—a core element of survival. Throughout the ages, nurses male and female have participated in healing practices to get people well, provided care to bring people back to health, and were instrumental in saving lives. These nursing practices have made a difference in the lives of people, their family, community, and society. The core of nursing then is to assist people in achieving balance to promote survival. This is achieved through the nursing process.

The nursing process entails nurse-to—client interactions. In this day and age of high-tech-low—touch, that direct interaction is losing ground. The client becomes a set of numbers on a monitor, a set of data to be analyzed, results of a laboratory test. The patient becomes an entity defined by finite information. Nursing process brings the nurse and client back together, to establish a human relationship. The nurse gets to find out from the patient what things upset their lives, their balance. Scientific evidence in the form of indicators help assess what causes those imbalances to help the nurse restore their health, maintain it, and prevent risks so that they can live in a more balanced way. Helping clients modify or change their behavior to balance—seeking could make a difference in their lives and their future. This is where nurses can find the greatest satisfaction in their profession.

Like all members of the helping profession, nurses have the ethical, moral, and legal obligation to provide care to anyone in need of assistance. Firemen rescue people out of burning buildings regardless of who they are. Police officers ensure the safety of the public they serve. Doctors save lives around the world. Nurses provide care to "all those committed to her keeping", part of the Florence Nightingale Pledge. A humanistic, caring approach to nursing, helping people find balance and health are basic human services. Nurses are found all over the world—taking care of people, one client at a time.

We know that we are all products of our culture. Everyone lives within a culture regardless of what it is, and to what ethnicity you belong. Both the nurse and the client are part of their cultures and are influenced by it. They bring these to the nurse-client interaction consciously or subconsciously. Using cultural data as part and parcel of assessment in the nursing process is essential in providing holistic and individualized care to all patients regardless of race, color, language, national origin, and gender. Balance is imbedded in cultural beliefs of people all over the world. I made it a point to focus on the influence of culture on human behavior as a chapter in the book. Examples of these cultural beliefs and practices as written by those who belong to that culture were included. By being aware and sensitive to each other's cultural beliefs, nurse-client communication and relationship are enhanced. This ultimately results in better outcomes.

I found that balance has a multitude of dimensions in human behavior. Studies of human behavior reveal that it is affected by both the internal and external environment. Balance is manifested only by behaviors that are observable, describable and measureable. The internal structures, processes and chemical compositions inside the human body are interrelated and controlled by our highly developed human brain. These serve as the internal impetus to maintain balance inside our body. But humans are also permeable to outside influences—the forces of nature, the elements surrounding us and our planet, our cultures, the organizations we built around us to make our lives more orderly, and even the stresses that our daily living and relationships produce. Human beings are viewed as systems that are affected by stimuli and produce behaviors as a human reaction to the multitude of inputs from our internal and external environments.

As I wrote the final chapter of this book, I felt that it was not really the end of my yearnings for balance in my own life. There is always something there beyond the hill. As a passage in one of my early poems, there is yet "another mountain to climb". Despite the science, balance seems to be just a place in my mind where I can find my zone of equilibrium—a place on top of the mountain where the air is rarified. I have to stop and enjoy the view—until I find another mountain to climb, with whatever energy and years I still have.

Daisy Magalit Rodriguez, MN, MPA, RN
San Ramon, California, USA

INTRODUCTION

Writing this book has been a challenging and a long journey of discovery for me. It began as a germ of an idea several years ago when I was still teaching in an associate degree nursing program south of the San Francisco Bay area. Over the next five years, I nurtured this idea but I did not quite know how to expand on this concept to turn it into a book. Paradoxically, the difficulty seemed to be in its seeming simplicity. There is no one definition that fits everyone's purpose. The word is so ubiquitous and part of everyday life that we take this concept for granted. It seems that you invariably encounter the word "balance" everywhere you turn. It is used in numerous instances and in a variety of subject matters. As a nurse, I have often encountered this term in health and illness concepts. But being a student of culture, I also come across this concept in studying various cultures. When I was studying physics and chemistry as a young university student, I was already introduced to the concept of balance. Balance is a basic concept in accounting, economics and politics. One cannot look at a work of art without being conscious of balance. And finding inner balance is key to mental health. These are but a few of the examples where the concept of balance is applied in everyday life. Could it be that there is a universality to this concept? Could it be an underlying concept in a view of life and the world in general? How do I relate it to what nurses do? How do I connect the dots?

The universality of balance: elements essential to survival

We know that forces and energies exist all around us. But I have often wondered, could there be other forces in the vastness of the universe—unseen, unperceived, and yet to be discovered by our intellect? And what about the products of the interactions of these forces—how do they affect us? What is the energy that gave birth to life and sustained it on this planet? Could this energy be balance? Is this energy tangible and how is it manifested? I perceived balance as a concept, an intangible idea. And yet you can feel, observe, measure, and describe its manifestations. These manifestations are in terms of behavior or activity of the organism, structure or system where it occurs. There appears to be a purpose to behavior and that is preservation of its existence. I began to think that behavior has a self-serving purpose: survival or maintenance of the integrity of the system to keep it whole and functioning.

As I developed a deeper understanding of balance, it led me to believe that balance in human beings does not exist in a vacuum. I looked at the elements that enable human beings to survive. The further I delved into my research, the more it became clearer that there are basic elements critical to survival. First, I looked at the definitions of balance—there are numerous. I found it in just about all branches of science and other fields of learning: physics, chemistry, mathematics, sociology, psychology, economics, geology, ecology, arts, and so on. I also came across terms that are used synonymously with balance: **equilibrium**, **harmony**, **symmetry**, **equality**, **stability**, etc. The one term that appears to be used more consistently is the concept of equilibrium—where two sides on a scale reach a point of equality. Positive cancels negative at the point of equilibrium. Stability is reached and ultimate balance is achieved. This, in my mind is the concept that best describes the element of balance. Applied to humans, a point of equilibrium is equal to stability, optimal health and well-being. Certainly, this concept is an essential element of balance.

I know as a nurse that the mechanism of **homeostasis** keeps the internal environment in a steady state of balance. Furthermore, I have always known as a nurse that health is critically important to life. Anything that jeopardizes life can lead to death. Therefore, **health** must be important to survival. I looked at the question of how humans survived throughout its history, depending only on themselves, their brains and their bodies to survive the harsh environment they lived in and travelled thousands of miles on earth. I chanced upon the concept of **adaptation** in my research in an old book on evolution. It said that the key to evolution is the concept of adaptation. Evolution and adaptation are not new terms. They have been around for a long time. But applied to the idea of balance and survival is something I have not come across. Certainly, in man's evolutionary process over eons of time, adaptation must have played a part in survival. We are what we are today because we have evolved and adapted to our environment.

Finally, the concept of **needs** as necessary for all human beings as a physical and psychological entity has been widely accepted. Abraham Maslow's Hierarchy of Needs has been a framework in many social science researches as well as nursing, and a basis for understanding human behavior. Needs have to be met for individuals, not simply to survive physically, but also to live a fulfilling life. The yearning for balance in their lives are met at various stages of this pyramid, influenced by factors such as developmental stage, personality, inherited traits, environmental conditions, and societal factors. People who are unable to find satisfaction of their needs remain in a state of imbalance—whether physically, or psychologically. To achieve a state of balance, the individual must find satisfaction of these needs in ways that are acceptable and appropriate within the society they live. Culture plays a major role in human behavior. It has a balancing effect on humans as a social being and part of a group. This becomes more obvious in the study of needs and the various realms of behavior. The need to achieve higher psychosocial levels appear to be part of human nature.

The achievement of the highest level—self-fulfillment, is where humans can find the fullest satisfaction in their lives as defined by themselves. The Maslow Hierarchy of Needs eventually became my model for my **Behavior Pyramid Model** delineating the various realms of behavior.

I identified the five elements of balance as: **adaptation, equilibrium, homeostasis, needs, and health**. Balance represents the convergence of those factors that all work synergistically for human survival. Related concepts that contribute to the totality of balance in human beings are: stability, symmetry, harmony, equality and well-being. I did not expand too much on these concepts in the book because I feel that these could be explored at another time. Suffice it to say that these related concepts are also reflections of balance and contribute to a deeper understanding of this concept. Arriving at the identification of the elements of balance was to me a major step in the book, but it was only the beginning. I had to expand on what these are and how they contribute to human survival. I felt like I was only looking at a prism with its various reflections. I had to look further into the mystery of balance and find some explanations on what it is, what affects it, and eventually, how I can bring it to the level of nursing practice. It seemed such a daunting task but I had to continue what I had already started. The hunger for answers kept nagging at my belly.

I have come to the conclusion that balance is the sum total of its elements—equilibrium, homeostasis, adaptation, needs and health. All these elements are interrelated and work in synchrony within the human system to enable it survive. And these elements are subject to influences from within the body and outside the body. These elements are those factors in the environments—internal and external. The body or organism has to have the capacity to respond to these influences through mechanisms that are innate. Behavioral responses can only happen if there is energy behind it—whether at the micro or cellular level, or the macro or organ/system level. Balancing influences must be present for that energy to exist. And the need to achieve balance seems to be innate. It is the body's "true north"—all the mechanisms and processes in human beings are directed towards survival and balance. Reaching for that highest level of balance and optimal health appears to be programmed in our brain—whether consciously or subconsciously.

That balance is part of the collective phenomenon of human existence reminds me of a car that cannot come to "life" without someone turning the ignition on. The car, as a modern human invention, is perhaps one of the greatest marvels of our time. But the intellect that Henry Ford possessed in conceptualizing, designing, and making that machine work did not occur in a vacuum. The collective thoughts and knowledge of human beings throughout the history of its existence gave rise to the creativity that enabled Ford to move this idea from conceptualization to execution. These knowledge and skills accumulated through human experiences throughout the ages are part of human development through evolutionary and adaptive processes. It became a way of life passed on from generation to generation. This way of life, called culture, was a tapestry woven throughout human existence.

The energy that makes the car run is derived from its fuel—gas or electricity. The car has to have all its parts in good working order and work interrelatedly with each other to contribute to the smooth functioning of the whole system. An integrated system of the mechanical parts of the car is necessary for it to function properly. Similarly, man is also a system that needs all its parts to work interrelatedly for it to function. But system alone does not explain the mystery of life and survival. The fuel provides the energy for the car to run. What similar energy is found in human beings that is required to "fire it up" and turn on the ignition of life? In studying the function of the cells in the human body, we find the basic key to that energy in the mitochondrion, a rod-like structure within the cell that functions as the main site for energy production. This energy is in the form of adenosine triphosphate (ATP) synthesized from foods ingested by the body. The cell uses this energy to perform the basic work necessary for cell survival and function. Without this energy, the cell runs out of fuel and dies. When cellular death occurs, the human being dies. Conditions of balance support cellular activity and function; without the existence of the elements of balance, cellular activity will come to a halt and life ceases.

I am convinced that balance in its various forms, is the common factor that exists in all human beings. By delving deeper into the meaning of balance, it became clear to me in my subsequent literature searches, that balance is the underlying concept of survival. This is the mantra of this book. It will be repeatedly emphasized throughout all the chapters. Balance has to be maintained by all human beings through its various elements in order to survive. Ultimately, the presence of balance explains why man is alive and continues to survive to this day. Balance, with its core elements of adaptation, homeostasis, equilibrium, needs, and health, are all essential to human existence and continued survival. How I arrived at the conclusion regarding these core elements was my first step into a journey of discovery that led me to the first chapter of the book.

I started with analyzing where balance occurs in a person's daily life. I looked at a typical example of a man (or woman) living in the present day world.

As man wakes up in the morning, gets out of bed, and starts walking to the bathroom, balance is set in motion. He needs a functioning neurological system in order to get up and walk with a balanced, steady gait. However, while he was still asleep, the internal environment of his body is being regulated automatically to maintain homeostasis, the internal self-regulating mechanism in the body to maintain physiologic balance. The fact that you have to eliminate body wastes, such as urine and feces are indications that his body continues to do its basic functions: sustain his life via physiologic maintenance of homeostatic balance within his body.

Then he proceeds through his day by getting behind the wheels of his car to go to work. His role in the family as the head and provider is something that his culture has dictated by tradition and practice. It is what makes him a productive member of society and gives him a sense of contribution to his family and community. It validates his sense of self-worth, which in turn boosts his self-esteem, feelings that contribute to his sense of well-being. He works for a manufacturing company, an organization that contributes to provide for the needs of the larger society. His income from his work in turn gives him the capability to perform his roles in the family and in the community. Success in his job and his profession will enable him to reach a stage of self-actualization, the highest level of need in Maslow's Hierarchy of Needs. He lives a healthy balanced life.

However, external and internal forces, the same ones that keep you healthy are the same ones that could conspire to tip the balance in the opposite direction: illness and disease. As he drives down the freeway, he notes that the traffic is getting heavier and heavier. An accident has caused a big traffic jam. He was getting late for work and begins to feel tense and stressed. Toxic fumes from the cars on the freeway assail his nostrils and increase the carbon dioxide level in his blood. Stress chemicals are released by the body producing stress responses. His muscles tense, his heart rate increases, his breathing becomes more rapid and his blood pressure starts to rise. Responding to stimuli from his external environment also sets in motion the processes of adaptation within his internal environment. If his body is unable to maintain balance by normalizing his blood pressure, heart rate and respirations, his homeostatic balance is upset and illness sets in.

Influence of the internal and external environments

The door to better understanding balance became wider as I began to understand that balance is affected by the internal and external environments of human beings. As we have seen from the example, internal balance is automatically maintained by innate mechanisms within the self-contained body of an organism. Cellular activity, as long as it has the energy to perform its functions will continue humming away, whether one is asleep or awake. The body functions as a coordinated system with parts, or organs, if you will, doing their own thing but all contributing to the total functioning of the organism. The control center of the human body is a well-developed brain and for some reason, much more superior than all other animals in the animal kingdom. This provided humans with the advantage to flourish by mastering their environment. Through their adaptive capabilities in the evolutionary process, they have been able to surmount untold obstacles that could have wiped them out from the surface of the earth long ago.

The elements in the external environment are numerous but can be grouped into the basic classifications of 1) nature (physical elements found in nature and as well as natural forces such as the sun, moon, the universe, air, water, gravitational forces, radiation, biological and chemical elements, etc., 2) culture (shared practices and beliefs passed on from generation to generation), 3) society (including family, community, organizations, governments, and groups of people), 4) technology (innovations, inventions, creative products used to improve human way of life). The external environment is also a source of stresses for people living in it. These stresses elicit physiologic responses that affect the human body. The manner that human beings deal with the external environment and internal impulses is manifested in their behavior.

Since man is influenced by both internal and external environmental factors, it stands to reason that it is permeable to those stimuli. An open system theory, first developed by the biologist Ludwig von Bertalanffy in the 1940's, was what I used to explain the concept of this permeability. The system model has been applied in many fields such as engineering, information technology, economics, politics, ecology, and so on. Man as an open system became one of my theoretical foundations in explaining the effects of the internal/external environments on behavior. The system theory was also a basis for the pioneering work of Betty Neuman in developing the Systems Model in nursing. Besides Maslow, other behavioral theories I used in this conceptualization are those of Pavlov, Freud, Erikson, Talcott Parson, and Bowen. Stress factors in the environment that affect behavior were also considered in the study of behavior and balance. Stress produces physiologic and psychosocial responses that disrupt balance. Its role in producing imbalances was considered important in the assessment of health.

Balance-seeking as a primary characteristic of human behavior is what I viewed as the result of that innate need to find balance in all human beings. The concept of balance-seeking is perhaps one of my brainstorms in this journey and an important step in the development of my thinking.

Behavior: unlocking balance elements

Behavior is a manifestation of activity of the human being. It can be measured, observed, and described. It is the key that unlocks the elements of balance already existing in human beings. Without behavior, balance cannot be manifested and actualized. The only way we know that balance exists is through behavioral manifestations—from the cellular level to the physical behavior of the person. Behavior is a projection of one's physical, mental, and emotional state—all ranges of human behavior. The individual's state of health is a manifestation of one's physical, mental, and psychosocial balance. This state of health is of utmost importance in health care. The factors that affect health include the sum total of internal and external environmental influences.

Behavioral theories guided my thinking in understanding the role of behavior in balance. They provided the theoretical foundations for the view I developed that behavior is balance-seeking to achieve the highest level of human psychosocial development. Maslow's Hierarchy of Needs was the basis for my Behavior Pyramid with four realms of behavior: 1) reflexive/automatic, 2) emotional/spiritual, 3) intellectual/rational, and 4) self-fulfillment levels. This follows the sequence of development of the brain in its evolution. The realms of behavior are manifested in subsets of balance-seeking behaviors. From a study of behavioral theories, I identified these subsets as manifestations of balance-seeking behaviors in the following areas: adaptive, physiologic/homeostatic, wellness, psychosocial (including personality systems, family systems and cultural practices), and physical behavior.

Culture and balance

The role of culture in human behavior is underscored in understanding balance. Imbedded in cultural beliefs are the concepts of balance and its opposite: **imbalance**. One cannot fully understand the concept of balance without understanding imbalance. This concept has long been understood and used by ancients in the dim past. The concept of balance is the concept of opposing forces—one that is also found in many cultures. This innate striving for balancing the effects of opposing forces as found in many other cultures are manifested as practices in religion, food and dietary practices, health and illness, birth and death, etc. Like the opposite sides of a weighing scale, balance will be tipped in the opposite direction if the forces of one side outweighs the other. The Asian culture in particular believes in the principle of "yin" and "yang" opposites: each side mirrors the other but viewed as a whole entity. This became part of their daily lives and an essential component of their belief systems. Health and illness attitudes, beliefs, and practices are of particular interest to me as a health care practitioner. I found that the concept of balance appeared to fit in with the goals of my nursing profession.

Health and well-being

As I developed the basic concept of balance, I started to realize how intimately related it is with health and well-being. One cannot exist without the other. I also realized that there are varying degrees of health and wellness, as well as varying degrees of illness. In the health care world, illness is an imbalance. Bringing the ill patient back to health is equivalent to bringing them back to a state of balance. I discovered the congruence between the concept of balance/imbalance and health care. Practitioners can practice within this frame of reference because this is exactly what we do—bringing patients back to a state of well-being and optimal health, a state of balance. Through interventions that are directed towards correcting the imbalances and helping patients change unhealthy or risky behaviors into healthy behaviors, then the goal of care is achieved.

The importance of health and well-being is a focus in this book because of its role in survival. No person can survive without health preservation. The goal of health professionals is to restore, preserve, and maintain health through their professional actions. This is what nursing wants to achieve—the optimal level of health possible for its clients. This is achievable through working with clients in supporting balance-seeking behaviors. Nursing is concerned with modifying and changing client behaviors in order to reach a level of health compatible with the client's values, beliefs, and attitudes. This is possible only with the client's acceptance of nursing interventions and teachings. Clients who are not engaged in balance-seeking behaviors are at risk for continued and worsening of their health problems, possibly progressing to worse levels of imbalances and ill health. Continued imbalances will eventually lead to death and/or disability. The key to this change is in the nurse-patient interaction during the nursing process. When nurses are able to make appropriate assessments, taking into consideration all the factors that impinge on the client's health status, including cultural influences, they are able to identify client's problems more accurately and hence an accurate nursing diagnosis leading to appropriate interventions.

Integrating Nursing Process

That the nursing process is an essential part in the determination of health status and state of balance of a client became very evident early on in my thinking in the writing of this book. This stems from the element of health in the concept of balance which is deemed essential for survival. The role of the nurse in health restoration, health preservation, and saving lives, has highlighted the central part nurses play in health care. The question of how the concept of balance connects with nursing is solved through the nursing process.

Nursing practice is based on knowledge, skills, and competence of the practitioner in nursing. Care is provided through an interaction with the client whether directly, or indirectly, on behalf of the client. This care is planned on the basis of information about the patient obtained through an assessment of relevant client data, identification of problems in client's response to problems, planning interventions, and evaluating response to the interventions. This process is called the nursing process, central to the professional practice of nursing.

Evidence-based practice starts with the gathering data through an assessment of the client that provides the basis for nursing actions. Similarly, nursing actions or interventions should also be based on scientific evidence to justify the rationale for interventions.

Development of the Balance Health Nursing Model

To this end, a nursing model of health was conceptualized and eventually developed using the concept of balance as the core concept. This is now called the **Balance Health Nursing Model** or **BHNM** as an acronym. Built around the balance concept is the health-illness continuum patterned after an accepted model of health and illness as a continuum. The commonly accepted definition of health by the World Health Organization was used as a basis for the concept of health. The model as proposed is not intended to replace but rather to augment the current models of nursing. The BHNM is an integrated approach, using current concepts in health and nursing, using the metaparadigm of nursing: person, health, environment and nursing. This model rests on the platform of the balance concept, integrating it into the total view of nursing and health.

It was necessary to establish a theoretical foundation for developing a model of nursing. The theories of Florence Nightingale (environment), Betty Neuman, (systems), Dorothy Johnson (behavioral systems), Sister Callista Roy (adaptation), Martha Rogers (unitary human beings), Margaret Newman (model of health), and Madeleine Leninger (culture), provided the theoretical "science" underpinnings of the balance model. Additionally, Jean Watson's Caring Theory was the underpinning of the "art" approach in nursing that is deemed inherent in the nursing process. Overall, using existing concepts and theories already developed by many scientists and thinkers from various diverse fields such as nursing, medicine, sociology, psychology, physiology, ecology, engineering, biological science, anthropology, physics, and chemistry, and the arts, an integrated model has emerged as the product of the evolution of my thinking.

The BHNM is where I have connected all the dots.

Balance Health Assessment Tool: An application of the BHNM

The real test of the model is in its applicability to the practice of nursing. I developed an Assessment Tool based on the balance/imbalance concept for use in health status assessment. Central to this tool is the nursing process starting with basic gathering of data about the patient. The nursing process is an organizing framework in nursing practice that involves the use of data gathering, identifying nursing diagnoses to describe the client's response to health problems, establishing goal and planning interventions, applying the interventions based on evidence, and evaluating the effects on the client's behaviors. The goal of the nursing process in the BHNM is consistent with the overall goal of nursing: changing and/or influencing client's response to identified nursing problems to produce positive outcomes using a holistic approach. This outcome is a state of balance in the physical, physiologic, and psychosocial status of the person.

The Balance Health Assessment Tool is a data-gathering tool intended to assist in identifying imbalances in the client/patient using the body system approach to determine physical/physiologic imbalances. Some information about the client's health behavior patterns will also be gathered to obtain a general idea of the patient's balance-seeking behavior patterns. Cultural data are also included as an essential aspect of overall client response to health problems and their ways of coping. A sample case study was included to illustrate the use of this tool. The assessment tool is the first step in designing an individualized nursing care plan for the client by health practitioners as well as nursing students in the health care setting.

Finally, it is the author's hope that this endeavor will help find focus in some of the major problems in health care today—health care disparities, caring for the burgeoning older adult population, and the unique problems of minority populations in the United States. By using the balance approach, we may start to realize again that there is a common thread that binds humanity. The survival of the human race depends on continuing the evolutionary link that allowed us all to withstand the test of time. Balance is that link that we need to preserve to maintain our survival on this planet. Nurses, as the keepers of the art and science of caring and healing, need to incorporate the concept of balance in their care to preserve its legacy for the next generations to come.

Book highlights

The book is divided into two parts:

1) Part I: Understanding balance
2) Part II: Balance in health and nursing:

Part I delves into the basic and overall understanding of the concept of balance and its basic elements: adaptation, homeostasis, equilibrium, needs, and health. It includes the role of the environment, behavior, and culture. Environment at the micro and macro levels are discussed as important to understanding balance. Similarly, behavior as balance-seeking is an important concept in understanding balance in human beings. It was necessary to include a chapter on the subsets of balance-seeking behavior to explain further how this is manifested in people's lives. Some theories are discussed to provide scientific evidence of the evolutionary thinking about behavior and related factors. Examples of the balance concept as part of cultural beliefs of many groups around the world were included to highlight the crucial influence of culture on people's behavior.

Part II discusses the relevance of balance in health and the nursing profession. It also includes some theoretical underpinnings of a balance concept in nursing and how it give rise to a model of balance and health. Nursing process is discussed as a component of the Nursing Process Balance model because it is important in the understanding of how nurses perform their functions and the centrality of this process. Nurses are part of the total environment of clients and also bring their own individuality to the nurse-patient interaction. The **Balance-Health Nursing Model (BHNM)** was developed based on all the concepts described in the book and represents a final confluence of these ideas. An Assessment Tool for health status as part of the data-gathering in the nursing process was developed and applied to a sample case study with emphasis on the cultural component.

The implications and challenges for the future in relation to changing global perspectives in health, health disparities, and care of the older adults are discussed in the afterword. The tantalizing question of balance as part of natural laws that govern the existence of human beings was raised. This is a subject that needs to be perhaps further explored by others, as we look more closely to try to understand the whole kaleidoscope of life on earth.

PART I

UNDERSTANDING BALANCE

Chapter 1

THE UNIVERSALITY OF BALANCE

"Mathematics expresses values that reflect the cosmos, including orderliness, balance, harmony, logic and abstract beauty."
—Deepak Chopra

"Physics depends on a universe infinitely centered on an equals sign."
—Mark Z. Danielewski, *House of Leaves*

Evidence that balance exists is everywhere. Achievement of balance is innate and necessary for human beings to survive. It is universal and inherent in all human beings. Without balance of those elements both internal and external to the human being, the human race may not have existed and continue to survive. It is the universality of balance that pervades all aspects of life and supports human beings in maintaining existence from the cellular level to the highest levels of human endeavors. Balance underlies all internal and external responses that enable human beings to continue to survive in its inexorable march through evolution.

BALANCE CORE ELEMENTS

In this book, this universality is contained in the interrelated core elements of balance, working synergistically, that enable all human beings to survive: **homeostasis, adaptation, equilibrium, needs, and health**. These terms will be mentioned throughout this chapter to lay the groundwork for the *concept of balance as the foundation of human survival*. Balance and the synergy of its elements, are at the core of life of human beings on this planet. Without continuous interrelationships and synchrony of these elements, in dynamic interplay between the factors in the internal and external environments of all human beings, imbalance will result, leading to death. Without balance, the human race is doomed for extinction.

The concept of balance intersects many fields in the modern present-day world. It appears in numerous publications in scientific fields of study, like a common thread within these sciences. Scientific principles have been used to understand human behavior both as an individual and as a member of society. Application of the concept of balance in understanding human nature and behavior is, not only necessary, but also inevitable.

Balance is a phenomenon that have existed in many different ways throughout human existence since time immemorial but has not been singularly defined as one concept. It is like looking at a prism with a multitude of facets but comes from one source. Balance is defined differently according to the perspective of the person defining it. To a physicist, balance means differently from what it means to an accountant, a chemist, mathematician, physiologist, nutritionist, sociologist, artist, or a biologist. These many perspectives lead to confusion and lack of uniformity in the definition of balance.

BALANCE DEFINED

Balance is referred to in this book within its broadest meaning encompassing its core elements in human beings of homeostasis, adaptation, equilibrium, needs and health, as well as its related concepts of harmony, stability, equality, symmetry and well-being. Discussion of core elements of balance and their related concepts will be discussed further in another chapter.

There are numerous definitions of balance within the context of the sciences, economics, art, health, accounting, culture, religion, nature and society. A dictionary definition of balance is "an instrument for weighing, esp. one with two matched hanging scales; a state of *equilibrium* in weight, value, etc; bodily equilibrium; mental or emotional *stability*; *harmonious* proportion of elements in a design, etc.; a weight, value, etc. that *counteracts* another; equality of debits and credits, or the difference between them.[1]

Other definitions include the following[2] 1. a weighing device, especially one consisting of a rigid beam horizontally suspended by a low—friction support at its center, with identical weighing pans hung at either end, one of which hold an unknown weight while the effective weight in the other is increased by known amounts until the beam is level and motionless; 2) a state of equilibrium or partly characterized by cancellation of all forces by equal opposing forces; 3) the power or means to decide; 4) state of bodily equilibrium or the ability to maintain bodily equilibrium; 5) a stable mental or psychological state; emotional stability; 6) a harmonious or satisfying arrangement or proportion of parts or elements, as in a design; 7) an influence or force tending to produce equilibrium; counterpoise; 8) the difference in magnitude between opposing forces or influences; 9) In Accounting: a) equality of totals in the debit and credit sides of an account; b) the difference between such totals, either on the credit or the debit side; 10) something that is left over; a reminder; 11. In Chemistry: equality of mass and net electric charge of reacting species on each side of an equation; 12) Mathematics: equality with respect to the net number of reduced symbolic quantities on each side of an equation; 13) a balance wheel.

The concept of balance has been used extensively in the physical sciences and other fields: (see Table 1).

The science of physics has used the fundamental principle of balance and equilibrium in weighing instruments, measurement of forces, gravity, energy, mechanics, thermodynamics, and motion studies. Isaac Newton,[26] considered the founder of modern physics in the seventeenth century, developed his three famous laws of motion on force and motion. His Law of Universal Gravitation explained the attraction of all objects on earth, as well as the planets in the universe, with each other. According to Newton, the force of gravity depends on mass and distance of objects from one another. It is the same law that governs movements of human beings, whether they are conscious of it or not. This universal force of gravity need to be balanced in order to maintain a state of stability in the planetary system, including our planet earth. These forces affect all inhabitants of the earth since time immemorial. Lacking a real understanding of these forces, early humans tried to explain and respond to these unseen, but perhaps intuitively felt, influences in ways their instincts dictated. As humanity diversified in innumerable ways, so did the forms in which they expressed these instincts—physically, psychologically, emotionally, socially, artistically, and spiritually.

In chemistry, the concept is applied in the movement of ions and molecules to balance electrical charges of reactants on both sides of the chemical equation. Mathematical principles in Algebra deal with equality of values on both sides of an equation. Algebra is a branch of mathematics where certain kinds of problems are solved using equations. An equation can be looked upon as a weighing scale or beam balance. Instead of a fulcrum, an equal (=) sign is used. This symbolizes that the values on each side are equal to each other. The concepts of mathematics as a science have been taught since the early childhood in schools as essential foundations of learning, as much as reading and writing.

It is also used as a concept in accounting and economics to bring the debit and credits sides into balance. In design, engineering and architecture, this concept has been used to create structures, buildings, and other habitations to create balance, stability and equilibrium within the system. Arts and design use related concepts of balance such as symmetry, harmony, and poise.

Ecology uses this concept in understanding the balance of nature. Biological science has been able to explain many of natural processes, such as homeostasis, nitrogen balance, and adaptation to create steadiness and stability in the organism. The study of anatomy and physiology, the cornerstone of medical science, is based on maintaining balance and equilibrium in the human body. Nursing uses holistic principles of balance to achieve physical, physiologic, and psychosocial balance in their clients. The fields of psychology and sociology uses concepts synonymous with balance such as harmony, equality, fairness, stability, composure, poise, calmness, and parity.

Whether used as a noun or verb, it denotes common concepts such as equilibrium, homeostasis, stability, counterbalance, order, compensation, harmony, symmetry, steadiness, counterbalance, proportion, counterpoise, and equality. It is clear that there is no one definition of balance. Different perspectives define it according to their frame of reference. This concept has been used in the sciences; other fields of human endeavor have used this concept to explain many phenomena that they have observed in nature and the universe. It is imbedded in healing beliefs in most cultures in the world. It could be said that this concept has pervaded all facets of human existence that dates back even before the dawn of civilization. Many modern inventions and innovations are based on the principle of balance.

The many definitions imply that there are numerous ways that balance is experienced by human beings. It could be compared to looking at a piece of crystal reflecting different colors when light is shown on it. Balance is a concept that could be looked at and experienced through the different prisms of each individual or group. In the human existence, it is experienced within the human body from the cellular level to the highest level of functioning in the brain and described in various ways. Physiologically, it is experienced as homeostasis at the cellular and body systems level; psychologically, it is felt as a mental and emotional well-being, as well as harmony with its surroundings with those elements outside of his physical being; aesthetically, it is expressed in the appreciation for balance in the arts as symmetry; and physically, the concept is applied in the physical sciences in the making and development of those materials and technologies throughout human history that man used in order to make his existence on this planet easier, that benefitted himself and others. These are all innate needs universally possessed by human beings. It is in human nature to seek to fulfill these needs.

References to balance are found in literatures, both scholarly and mundane. The term has become so commonplace and used in different contexts in daily life. It appears to be a basic underlying concept that cuts across all races, languages, ethnic origin, gender, culture, religions, health practices, socioeconomic status, and geographic locations. The concept became imbedded in many different ways in how people deal with everyday living. Balance and health have been intricately connected because of its common denominator of life preservation. To preserve health is to promote survival.

Given the various definitions of balance, it is the intent of the author to use the term within the scope of human experience and the critical role it plays in human survival. The concept applies to all areas of existence—from the most basic needs to man's highest aspirations. It is not a static state but a dynamic interplay of all the forces that impinge on the individual, both internal and external. It is both the process and product of the dynamic interrelationships of opposing forces of life's most basic elements: adaptation, homeostasis, equilibrium, needs and health. Balance defined in this book, is ***the dynamic interplay of all forces that equalize each other within the internal and external environments of a person"***.

SURVIVAL AND EVOLUTION

Despite advanced knowledge in the modern world and the advent of the internet where information is easily accessible through computers, no one knows for sure exactly when life began on this planet. Without hard scientific evidence that can be obtained at present from the earth's billions of years of history, one can only surmise that balance existed with the first spark of life in the universe. The balance of environmental conditions that existed eons of years ago in the origin of our world presumably became conducive to the survival of the first biologic organisms. It can be inferred that life on earth began with the balancing of forces of the external environment: the heat of the sun balanced with the coolness of the night, the balance of the amount of oxygen and other elements that support life, presence of life-giving water, nutrients that sustained human beings in their primeval lives, dealing with the forces of the environment that threatened their safety, etc. Gravitational forces that affect all objects on earth also influence man's existence.

In evolutionary terms, man is relatively new as a biologic being in the world. Archaeologists digging through the debris of thousands of centuries have started to uncover the complicated history of man's evolution. A recent find in South Africa appeared to have discovered the roots of the first humans which date back only sometime between three million and two million years ago[3]—a relatively new development in the history of the earth, or the universe, for that matter. But while the biologic remains of the first fossil sea animals date from about six hundred million years ago, it was only about 345 million years ago when the precursors of land-dwelling creatures began to appear in the form of reptiles. These terrestrial forms of life are mammals. Man is a mammal who succeeded the reptiles in the evolutionary process. According to research data, primates, the main subgroup of mammals to which man belongs, first appeared about sixty-five million years ago. Features of primates, such as a large brain and good vision enabled them to explore and manipulate their environment. As time went on, man developed a larger brain and the capacity for higher level thinking that enabled him to adapt and survive as a species. More than any other mammal, man evolved as better able to adapt to and control his environment. Key to man's continued survival and development as a species is the process of ***adaptation.***[4]

How man was able to make the quantum leap from being an animal to an intelligent human being is yet to be discovered and continues to be an area of controversy even in this day and age of advanced scientific knowledge. The religious view that man is a creation of a Supreme Being is neither disputed nor affirmed in this book. This is rather a matter of individual belief and outside the scope of this book.

ADAPTATION IN HUMAN SURVIVAL

The human anatomy evolved as an adaptive development. Adaptation is the process by which all living creatures on earth modify themselves through many generations to take advantage of their environment and in so doing ensure their survival.[4] Of all the creatures on earth, man appeared have been the best able to adapt to changing conditions in the environment over time and develop fully into intelligent beings. From their primeval beginnings throughout the process of evolution, man had inherited and developed those characteristics that were adaptive. One example of adaptation is the bipedal, or two-legged striding gait, which was different from its ancestors, the first primates, that appeared about sixty-five million years ago. This freed his hands to manipulate the surroundings and develop tools necessary for his existence. This also enabled him to run and deal with obstacles in order to escape from predatory wild animals and adverse environmental conditions.

From the moment that the first humans began to walk upright his primeval brain possessed the anatomic structure, the *cerebellum*, to enable him to maintain his balance walking on two legs, not four, as his forbears did. This structure, called the "little brain"[5] contains over 50% of the total number of neurons in the brain. With input from sensory apparatus in the inner ear, it is important in making postural adjustments for the body to maintain physical balance. Sensory inputs are processed by higher centers of the brain which are then integrated by the cerebellum so that the necessary muscular activities are executed smoothly. These movements are manifested as observable behaviors. The smooth walking gait of a human being, and other motions are products of a complex coordination of the sensory and motor functions of the brain.

Other human characteristics developed over time to adapt to the constantly changing environment. As scientists pieced together the history of man's development, they were able to come to conclusions that pointed to adaptation as the process that enabled human beings to survive and thrive as a species, while other less-adapted animals followed the way of extinction. Charles Darwin, the famous English naturalist in the 19th century, called this the process of natural selection, his basic mechanism of evolution. Man's intellect, directly associated with an increase in size of the brain, and increased acuity of his sensory apparatuses enabled him to deal more effectively with the world around him. Largely contributory to this adaptation was his ability use his hands, having evolved into a bipedal animal, that eventually enabled man to develop advanced tools. The dawn of modern civilization was heralded by such crude beginnings.

HOMEOSTASIS: INTERNAL REGULATION

Existence of the biologic organism, from which man eventually evolved, depended on the continuous balance of those external and internal factors to propagate life on this planet as it still does. In the continuing process of evolution, man must continually respond, react and adapt to stimuli both internally and externally to ensure his survival on the planet. Internal processes within the body of the organism operate to maintain life. These internal processes are called ***homeostasis,*** defined as "the state of dynamic equilibrium of the internal environment of the body that is maintained by the ever-changing processes of feedback and regulation in response to external or internal changes".[6] It is the state of equilibrium in the internal environment of the body maintained by adaptive responses that promote healthy survival. The goal of homeostasis is to restore and maintain internal balance, stability, health, and well-being of the individual.

Homeostasis starts at the cellular level and controlled by the higher functions of the brain through hormonal regulations. A vast array of chemical changes happen within or outside the cell in response to stimuli in the internal and/or external environment of the body. Each cell in the human body performs a function that contributes to the overall functioning of the entire body. The human cell is like a small factory—it takes in a continuous flow of raw materials for processing and processes its own chemical wastes for disposal. The continuous series of chemical changes that happen in and around the cells is what determines human life on this planet. Although cells are specialized in their functions, they must work harmoniously with other cells if the whole body is to function smoothly. The human body can only function efficiently when the equilibrium between the cells, tissues and organs is maintained. It is the concept of harmony and balance of all the different parts of the body that make it a living, breathing organism. Dysfunction of a cell or a group of cells disrupts this balance and leads to disease or disorder, or even death. Homeostatic regulation allows an organism to function effectively in a broad range of environmental conditions.

To maintain homeostasis, organisms have at least three interdependent components that enable it to regulate itself.[7,8] 1) the receptor which is the sensing component that monitors and responds to stimuli or changes in the environment, 2) a control center, which receives and processes the stimuli and determines the range within which equilibrium is maintained in the body, 3) the effector, which corrects any deviation from which the stimuli or change had created, thus allowing the organism to go back to its original state of dynamic stability. This involves both positive and negative feedback mechanisms. These mechanisms are either switched on or off depending on the presence or absence of a stimuli that changes the equilibrium of the body. This concept would be important in understanding human response and behavior to effect balance.

Homeostasis is also viewed as a property of a system that regulates the internal environment to maintain a stable and constant environment within the system. It works via feedback mechanisms in response to stimuli and regulated by chemicals released by various organs in the body. From a state of relative stability and equilibrium, a body reacts to stimuli that tends to disrupt or cause an imbalance in its normal functioning by activating a positive feedback mechanism. These are mechanisms that are designed to accelerate or enhance the output created by a stimulus that pushes levels out of normal ranges, or upsets the equilibrium. Once a certain threshold is reached, the body responds by diminishing the output via a negative feedback mechanism. This mechanism consists of processes that reduces the output or activity of any organ or system back to its normal range of functioning, thereby restoring stability and balance once more.

An example of this positive-negative feedback loop is the regulation of blood pressure. When the body sees a threat (stimulus), it responds by activating the sympathetic nervous system, thereby constricting blood vessels and increasing cardiac output to increase blood flow to the vital organs. This response raises the blood pressure and increases heart rate, a positive feedback. Blood vessels can instantly sense resistance of blood flow against the walls when blood pressure rises. The blood vessels, acting as receptors, relay this message to the brain. Presuming that the stimulus has been effectively neutralized, the brain in turn, sends a message to the heart and blood vessels which are the effectors. The heart rate decreases as the blood vessels increase its diameter (vasodilation). These changes cause the blood pressure to fall back to its normal range (a negative feedback).

The whole body is akin to an integrated system with internal feedback mechanisms of inputs and outputs so that it could maintain this internal balance. This state is when the body is able to regulate itself, heal itself, and fend off invasion of foreign elements that pose a risk to its integrity. For instance, the body's normal defenses, such as the immune system and the reticulo-endothelial system are in a state of readiness to respond to an internal threat but are not mobilized until the threat is actually present. When confronted with a threat, i.e. infection or inflammation, the body summons those defenses to fight off the foreign substances and repairs itself so that it will go back to its original state of stability.

Another example of internal regulation in human beings is the homeostatic regulation of body temperature. When the internal temperature becomes excessive due to external factors such heat from the sun on a summer day, sweating is induced through these processes in order to cool down the body. Or in the winter when the body experiences excessive cold, the mechanisms that induce shivering to produce heat are set into motion. Maintaining his body temperature within levels conducive to comfort and safety, another basic need, is a function of both internal regulating mechanisms and manipulation of the external environment.

EQUILIBRIUM

In common parlance, balance and equilibrium are used synonymously. However, the author would like to draw a distinction between the two concepts in this book to avoid confusion. Balance is used as a term to denote a broader scope that encompasses other concepts, such as equilibrium. Equilibrium also has various meanings, depending on the context it is used.

A common definition of equilibrium is "a stable condition in which forces cancel each other".[9] Other definitions of equilibrium are in the context of the field of science or study where it applies. Some definitions of equilibrium are: 1.Psychology/Mental Health: a state of feeling or mental balance; 2) thermodynamic equilibrium: any unchanging condition or state of a body, system, resulting from the balance or cancelling out of the influences or processes to which it is subjected; 3) physics: a state of rest or uniform motion in which there is no resultant force on a body; 4) chemistry: the condition existing when a chemical reaction and its reverse reaction takes place at equal rates; 5) physiology: a state of bodily balance, maintained primarily by special receptors in the inner ear; 6) economics: the economic condition in which there is neither excess demand nor excess supply in the market[9] Synonyms for equilibrium are equipoise, steadiness, stability.

Numerous terminologies related to equilibrium and its related concepts are found in literatures under many subject matters and disciplines such as physics, chemistry, biology, physiology, ecology, and economics. The following are examples: [27]

Biology:

Equilibrioception is the sense of a *balance* present in human beings and other animals.
Genetic equilibrium is a theoretical state in which a population is not evolving.
Homeostasis is the ability of an open system, especially living organisms, to regulate its internal environment (mentioned elsewhere in the chapter).

Physics

> *Hydrostatic equilibrium* is the state of a system in which compression due to gravity is *balanced* by a pressure gradient force.
> *Mechanical equilibrium* is the state in which the sum of the forces, and torque, on each particle of the system is zero.
> *Radiative equilibrium* is the state where the energy radiated is balanced by the energy absorbed.
> *Thermal equilibrium* is a state where an object and its surroundings cease to exchange energy in the form of heat, i.e. they are at the same temperature.

Chemistry

> *Chemical equilibrium* is the state in which the concentrations of the reactants and products have no net change over time.
> *Diffusion equilibrium* is when the concentrations of the diffusing substance in the two compartments are *equal*.
> *Solubility equilibrium* is any chemical *equilibrium* between solid and dissolved states of a compound at saturation.
> *Thermodynamic equilibrium* is the state of a thermodynamic system which is in thermal, mechanical, and chemical *equilibrium*.

Economics

> *Economic equilibrium* is a condition (of stability) in economics.
> *Equilibrium price* is the price at which quantity supplied equals quantity demanded.
> *Static equilibrium*, is the intersection of supply and demand in any market.

Sociology

> *Social equilibrium* is a system in which there is a dynamic working balance among its interdependent parts.

Ecology

> Balance of Nature—based on the theory that ecological systems are usually in a stable equilibrium.

These related concepts of equilibrium appear to suggest that: 1) there is an existence of opposing elements, forces, or energy within a system; 2) it involves a dynamic interplay of these forces; and 3) a state of relative stability is achieved when forces balance each other in the system.

In the human body, it is the state wherein the body is able to maintain the parameters between factors that promote normalcy and balance, and those that cause abnormality and imbalance. This is achieved through the mechanisms of homeostasis, the self-regulating mechanism of the body to maintain internal equilibrium. So long as the body performs its functions normally and keeps those elements necessary to sustain life within a range of equilibrium (range of normal values), the body is in a state of stability. Each unit or body organ system does its function to contribute to the functioning of the total whole. The body maintains a range within which it is able to sustain the health and well-being of the individual. These ranges are values that have been identified as falling within the continuum of normalcy (i.e. normal values for cholesterol: adult/elderly (150-200 mg/dL); child (120-200 mg/dL); infant (70-175 mg/dL); newborn (53-135 mg/dL).[10] These are the results of tests performed in laboratories and widely accepted as normal findings. Results that fall outside of these ranges are considered abnormal. A state of abnormality is one that is not in balance and could cause disease or disorder in the body system affected. Restoration of equilibrium would entail correcting the abnormality leading back to a state of balance or equilibrium.

The balance scale has been identified mostly as the physical representation of the concept of equilibrium. It is this symbol that has persisted throughout the pages of human history. Symbols of balance have been used since the ancient times. Libra, the seventh sign of the zodiac was represented by the scales, symbolizing the principle of symmetry and balance. In Roman mythology, Libra is depicted by the symbol of the scales held by Astraea (also known as Virgo), the goddess of justice.[11]

Sometime during man's earlier history, an instrument for determining weight was invented. It is typically designed with a bar and a fulcrum at the center. The *fulcrum*, or the middle point is where this equilibrium occurs. From one end of the instrument is suspended a scale with a known weight, and the other holding the object to be weighed. The value of the object is determined when a balance is achieved between the two sides of the fulcrum. For balance to exist, there must be at least two opposing forces that serve to equalize each other's values. Anything that outweighs one side will disturb this balance and will tip it towards the side with the greater value or weight.

The concept of balance using a weighing scale instrument has existed for thousands of years. The oldest evidence of using the weighing scale for determining absolute weights dates back to between 2400 and 1800 B.C.E. in the Indus River valley, now modern-day Pakistan. The ancient Egyptians are thought to have developed the first known weighing instruments, which they probably used to measure gold. Ancient hieroglyphic symbol for gold found in archaeological finds indicated the use of these scales perhaps for this purpose.[12,13]

Over time, the weighing scale has come to symbolize balance of two values of which one counteracts the other to produce a state of equilibrium, stability or equality. It also denotes states of harmony, symmetry, neutrality or steadiness. What was probably intuitively sensed by human beings since the beginning of their existence found expression in the instruments that they used to survive and thrive. Long before evidence of such inventions were discovered, humans that walked the earth and started using their intellect perhaps became conscious of the energy that enabled them to maintain their very existence. Already hard-wired In their brain to maintain their equilibrium and balance to walk upright, man perhaps was able to intuitively sense the need to maintain balance. This may have found expression in the instruments that they created to make the challenges of their daily existence easier. Balancing the forces of their external environment with their instinct for survival and balance probably had provided them with a sense of kinship with their environment. For instance, the Navajo American Indians, through their ancient heritage, have retained the belief that it is essential for man to live *in harmony* with nature and its elements.[14]

IMBALANCE: A STATE OF DISEQUILIBRIUM

If one is to think of the concept of balance as a scale, with balance on one side and imbalance on the opposite side, it is easy to visualize why these are two opposing but self-balancing forces.

DIAGRAM I.1 DYNAMICS OF BALANCE AND IMBALANCE

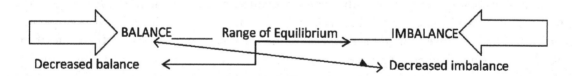

The diagram of the dynamics of balance and imbalance is illustrated above. Imbalance cancels the effects of balance and renders it unequal. A weighing scale with two equal values on each side will be in perfect equilibrium. Adding extra weight on one side will tip the balance towards the side that has the greater weight. This will negate the balancing effect and hence render it unbalanced. In order to restore balance, an adjustment needs to be made so that both sides will be restored to its former state of equilibrium. Similarly, the body in a normal state of balance, becomes imbalanced or falls outside the normal range of equilibrium.

In order to return to its normal state of balance, an adjustment needs to be made. Hence, decreasing balance will lead to imbalance, decreasing imbalance will lead back to balance. Balance-seeking forces will tend to move towards equilibrium.

HUMAN NEEDS : MASLOW'S HIERARCHY

A **need** is something required or essential.[15] According to a model developed by **Abraham Maslow** in the 1940s, all human beings have needs that have to be fulfilled which he arranged in a hierarchy. The basic needs necessary for survival take priority over any other need. These basic needs are physiologic which include oxygen, water, food, shelter, elimination, and sexuality. Other human needs also exist, such as the needs for: safety and security, love and belongingness, esteem, and self-actualization—the highest level attainable for human beings. Various researchers have used Maslow's model of human behaviors as a basis for their studies. Different terminologies have been used to describe the five levels of Maslow's hierarchy. However, these five levels have basically been recognized and cited in many publications:[16]

These needs are arranged in a hierarchy with the most basic physiological needs at the bottom and the highest level, self-actualization, at the top. This hierarchy of needs is commonly represented as a pyramid. The more basic needs have to be met first before higher needs take precedence. Maslow believed that an individual's behavior is influenced by the individual's attempt to meet his needs. [17,18] Meeting his basic needs, such as accessing food and water required him to deal with the external environment. He had to actively seek those elements that the body required for life-giving sustenance. These needs that required to be fulfilled or met are physiologically driven, which man was equipped by nature to ensure his survival. Unmet physiologic needs however, lead to deprivation, a state of imbalance. Unless man did something to meet these needs and restore his physiologic balance, man would die. Extinction of the human race was certainly not one of the options that nature intended.

Physiologic needs such as air, water and food, are the most potent of all other needs—these have to be met to ensure human survival. These needs are what drive humans' instincts for survival. Homeostasis is what maintains balance of elements and fluids in the internal environment of the human body. Once physiologic needs are relatively satisfied, the needs for safety and security then take precedence.

Safety and security could take various forms such as a need for stability, protection, security, freedom from threat or aggression, and external threats such as calamities, natural disasters, wars, violence, or trauma. A feeling of lack of security could arise from financial and economic crisis, such as loss of job or demotion. Loss of an important family member who provides support for the family can affect a person's sense of security. Children and young people may feel the effects of threats to physical safety more than adults.

Love and belonging, the third layer human needs, is related to the social nature of man. This need is met through interaction with other people, especially those whom the individual feels are most important in his/her life. The need for affection is necessary for humans to feel a sense of belonging and acceptance. This could come from within the family, friends, or from social groups such as organizations, clubs, office, gangs, and other social connections. Being part of the same ethnic or cultural group can also give the person a sense of belonging as part of the community.

Esteem needs pertain to those needs for self-respect, self-esteem and self-worth. It is a normal human desire to be valued and respected by others. This gives rise to behaviors that contribute to the person's sense of value and contribution to activities participated in by others. Satisfaction of this need entails a healthy sense of self-respect and respect for others. In order to be valued by others, the person also has to recognize the value of others. Psychological imbalances can result from a low self-esteem. Inability to find a balance between one's need for recognition and acceptance by others with an appreciation of the worth of other people becomes an emotional imbalance.

Self-actualization is the level where a person is able to achieve his/her full potential and continues to realize this potential. It is the desire to become everything that one is capable of becoming. This could find expression in a multitude of forms and defined solely by the individual's sense of achievement. However, in order to reach the highest level, one must meet the previous levels from the lowest to the next levels: physiological, safety, love and esteem. This is the stage where the person achieves a complete state of balance and equilibrium in all aspects of life: physiologic, physical, mental, spiritual and emotional. In this context, a need is defined as "something that is lacking or deficient that is required or desired by the individual in order to fill a deficiency and achieve physical, psychological and mental well-being, leading to a state of equilibrium or balance".

HEALTH, WELLNESS, AND ILLNESS

The concept of balance is intimately connected with health. Many cultures believe that the basic functions of the body are related by bodily fluids or "humors". [19] A proper balance of these humors was necessary to maintain good health; an imbalance leads to illness. These health beliefs are deeply rooted in their cultures and have been passed on from generation to generation. Ancient healing traditions emanated from deeply held ideas about how the body is able to maintain balance and harmony both with the external world and within their bodies.

These practices are not far removed from present-day beliefs about health and illness. With new information, knowledge, and technology came various modes of health preservation and illness prevention. But the basic concept of balancing internal and external factors remain at the core of human health and wellness.

The **World Health Organization (WHO)** defines health as a "state of complete physical, mental and social well-being and not merely the absence of disease or infirmity".[20] This definition implies an optimum state of health which had not been changed since 1948 when the WHO constitution was signed on July 22, 1946 by representatives of 61 states and placed into effect on April 7, 1948.

The state of well-being varies from one individual to another and is variedly defined by each individual. Well-being is commonly defined as a condition or a state characterized by health, happiness, and prosperity. This state of well-being, according to the WHO definition encompasses physical, mental, and social aspects of the person. To achieve a state of well-being, a balance of these three dimensions must be achieved. The individual who lacks one aspect may compensate in another in order to achieve a balance.

Balance is therefore important in maintaining the well-being of an individual. How one achieves well-being and be in a state of health varies from one individual to another. Health as a state of being is defined by each person according to their own values, personality, health beliefs, and lifestyle. Being healthy may not necessarily mean the absence of a pathological condition. This suggests a view of health as influenced by factors that are more complex than the absence of disease.

It is therefore important to look at the concept of balance as more closely aligned with the WHO definition of health. Maintaining a balance of these three dimensions keeps the individual in a state of wellness or well-being. An imbalance in any of the three dimensions of health produces a decreased state of well-being. When this condition is left uncompensated or unadjusted, it will lead to a disturbance in the person's well-being. Decreased well-being is a state of illness. *Illness* is defined as a condition of being in poor health or presence of disease, or a disturbance in one's normal functioning.

Wellness and illness are opposing and complex concepts in health. These two concepts are core values in healthcare and are represented in the form of a continuum. The wellness/illness continuum is described as the range of an individual's total health. This continuum is dynamic and ever-changing and highly individual. It is influenced by the individual's physical condition, presence or absence of disease, mental health, and social well-being. Wellness on one end of the continuum is the state of optimal health, equilibrium, well-being, and balance; illness on the opposite side of the continuum is a state of dysfunction, disequilibrium, and imbalance. This diagram is a representation of the Wellness/Illness continuum that parallels the Balance/Imbalance continuum.

Wellness _____Range of Health_____ Illness

　　　　Optimal state of health　　　　　　　　　　Impaired state of health

BALANCE_____Range of Balance_____IMBALANCE

　　　　(balance, equilibrium, well-being)　　　　　(imbalance, disequilibrium, dysfunction)

DIAGRAM 1.2 : Wellness-Illness continuum and Balance-Imbalance continuum

The balance of these two states defines the level of health of the individual. Inability to maintain a state of wellness will lead to a state of illness; decreasing factors that cause illness will move the person towards the wellness side of the continuum. Total wellness is reached when an optimal state of balance and equilibrium is achieved by the individual.

Optimal health as the state of ultimate wellness is the goal of human existence. There are many factors that influence or affect the individual's state of optimal health, both internal and external. Internal factors include the body's ability to maintain a steady equilibrium of the body's physiologic function and processes or *homeostasis*, psychological state, personality traits, age, gender and genetic make-up. External factors include environmental influences such as temperature, environmental sanitation, weather, cultural influences, role of family, religion, and socio-economic factors. A disruption or imbalance in any or a combination of these factors can potentially lead to illness in any or all dimensions of health: physical, mental or social.

HUMAN BEHAVIOR AS BALANCE-SEEKING

Internal forces, or physiologic processes, that operate automatically inside the body like a well-oiled machine have existed since the beginnings of the biologic organism called man. But in order to exist at the level that man is able to balance the forces within himself and the forces outside of his physical self required ***balance-seeking behaviors***.

In the beginning of mankind, these behaviors were perhaps very primitive and limited to the satisfaction of his *basic need*s that met his requirements for survival. Without those balance-seeking behaviors, man would not have been able to protect himself from the harsh effects of environmental elements. For instance, building a shelter to shield himself from the heat of the sun or the cold of winter is a ***balance-seeking*** **behavior**. The concept of balance-seeking could then be defined at the very basic level as *actions carried out by an individual to satisfy unmet needs.* As basic human needs are met, other needs emerge beyond the primeval physiologic needs. Psychosocial needs take over and become more dominant in the person's behavior. Still, the urge to seek balance remains the underpinning of human behavior. It is the driving force that influences humans to strive more and more to achieve a sense of well-being and self-fulfillment in the highest order. In essence, this innate urge to seek balance is the fire that enables man to reach beyond his physiologic needs to go further and further into horizons of higher levels of relationships and aspirations never before explored. Other internal factors also influence individual behavior and responses such as biological variations, personality, race, gender, genetically inherited traits, developmental stage, perception of time and space, and intellectual capacity.

HUMAN BEING AS AN OPEN SYSTEM

Man's ability to survive and thrive on this planet relies on his ability to maintain internal balance and interact with the external environment. As a biologic being, man must adapt to forces and influences in his world that affect him directly or indirectly. His capacity to perceive, process, interpret and respond to stimuli is affected by numerous factors within a zone with boundaries that only the person can define. This zone is the system within which the individual moves and lives.

What is a system and what are its fundamental components? A system is a set of connected or interrelated parts forming a complex whole. The Systems Theory[21] was first proposed by biologist Ludwig von Bertalanffy in the 1940s and furthered by Ross Ashby in 1956. Systems concepts include system-environment boundary, input, output process, state, hierarchy, goal-directedness, and information. Applications of the Systems Theory are numerous— from information technology, engineering, economics, politics, ecology, management, organizational models and human behavior. A system can be open, holistic, or closed. Systems theory has also been applied in the study of human behavior. A main concept of the theory in human behavior is that persons are in continual relationship with their environment and systems tend towards equilibrium.[22]

An open system is one that interfaces and interacts with its environment by receiving inputs from and delivering outputs to the outside.[23] The open system possesses permeable or porous boundaries that permit the transmission of interaction and information across human physical and psychological boundaries. The porosity and permeability of human boundaries can only be individually defined. Human beings are open systems and by having the ability to allow inputs from the outside, process this input within the body and produce outputs in terms of behavior, the human being is able to adapt quickly to the changes in the external and internal environment. By allowing the flow of inputs/stimuli into its boundaries as well as the delivery of outputs to the outside, the human system is able to adapt to constant changes, thereby improving its probability of survival.

The outputs delivered to the outside are measured in terms of directly observable human behavior and will be explained in a later chapter. These behaviors are executed in four realms that closely approximate Maslow's Hierarchy of Needs Pyramid: 1. Reflexive or automatic, 2) Emotional/Spiritual, 3) Rational/Intellectual, and 4) Self-fulfillment

While the System Theory is useful in the study of the place of man in the context of the world around him by looking at individual parts, it is necessary to view the human being as a whole entity and not just the sum of its individual parts. The human being is much more complicated than just the numeric sum of its parts. The holistic view of individual persons is the best approach in understanding the complexity of man.

A **holistic** view of a system is an approach that is more integrative and considers the integrity and function of the whole organism.[24] Holism's view is that the system should be viewed in its entirety rather than its individual parts. Besides ensuring the integrity of the individual parts, the total functioning of the whole is the ultimate goal. It is like making sure that all the parts of the car engine are intact, well-oiled and working properly. A missing part could damage the entire system and not make the engine run.

Similarly, the human body cannot function properly if one system is malfunctioning. For instance, failure of the heart to pump blood efficiently to the rest of the body, in the case of congestive heart failure, will affect other systems of the body and put the body in a state of imbalance. Outside conditions could exacerbate heart failure, such as extremes in temperatures. Emotional stresses in the family could also contribute to heart failure. By treating the client holistically, better outcomes (outputs) may result.

RELATED CONCEPTS: SYMMETRY, HARMONY, STABILITY, EQUALITY, AND WELL-BEING

Symmetry

Balance or beauty of form resulting from balance is a definition of symmetry. Other words synonymous with symmetry are: proportion, equality, harmony, equilibrium, and equivalence It is the property that describes an equality or balance of an object or subject on each side. Symmetry is found in the human body, nature, and the arts. The human body is generally born with each side in symmetrical proportion i.e., left side appears the same as the other side on the outside. Internally, most of organs are also arranged symmetrically. Except for single organs such as the heart, stomach, liver, pancreas, many internal organs are duplicated on each side of the body. Hence, human beings are born with two arms and legs, two lungs, two kidneys, even two hemispheres of the brain. The opposite of symmetry is asymmetry, an imbalance.

Symmetry is found in the arts such as architecture, painting, sculpture and interior decoration. It is a sense of balance perceived by the individual through his/her senses that provokes a pleasing sensation, a sense of balance, harmony and equilibrium. An object of art with symmetry evokes a feeling of order and balance that may differ from one individual to another. As humans evolve into more complex beings with a greater sense and appreciation of the world around them, the sense of balance becomes more appealing to their loftier needs. Asymmetry evokes a sense of imbalance, chaos and disorder. These two concepts probably found its way in their creative expressions.

Harmony

It is a term generally used to signify a blending of elements that are sensed as pleasing to the individual. In music, it is unity of musical patterns that creates a sensation of accord, rhythm and melody. Man also seeks harmony with the world within which he lives by finding a sense of balance with nature and its elements. Harmony in interpersonal relationships is also one of the values of human beings. This finds expression in certain religions and cultural beliefs. For instance, in the American Indian culture, man and nature are intimately intertwined. Being in total harmony with nature underlies their belief systems. To be in harmony with nature is to respect it in the same manner as they respect their body. Nature is their source of life and they must have a harmonious relationship with it to maintain a peaceful existence.

Harmony is also an underpinning in religious teachings in some Asian American populations such as Buddhism, Confucianism and Taoism.[25] Buddhism teaches harmony or non-confrontation expressed in such moderations in behavior as self-discipline, patience, humility, selflessness, dedication, modesty and friendliness. The core belief of Confucianism is humanism. It teaches achievement of harmony through its relationship with society embodied in **ren**, **yi,** and **li**. *Ren* is an obligation of altruism and humaneness for other individuals within a community, *yi* is the upholding of righteousness and the moral disposition to do good, and *li* is a system of norms and propriety that determines how a person should properly act within a community. *Taoism* teaches harmony between humans and nature. A principle of Taoism is the dynamic balance between man and nature.

Stability

The essence of equilibrium and balance is a state of stability, where the forces impinging on an object are not exerting energy toward or away from the center or fulcrum. A key concept in physics is Newton's Law of Universal Gravitation.[26] As the pull of earth's gravity keep objects relatively firmly planted on the earth's surface, all objects also exert a gravitational attraction on other objects. All objects on earth are made up of matter with its individual mass. Matters are made up of particles that are constantly in motion. All physical bodies are attracted to each other due to the force of gravity. Force is defined as a push or a pull. This force causes the body to move. The earth always exerts a force on all objects. Forces that are opposite in direction and equal in size or weight are called balanced forces. Forces that are not opposite and equal are called unbalanced forces. Balanced forces cause an object to remain at rest. This state of rest is a state of stability, where the net force exerted on opposite sides is zero.

Applied to the human body, stability is its natural tendency. To be unstable is to be unbalanced. Stability in the internal environment means a state of constancy where homeostasis is maintained. A stable state of mind denotes a constancy and balance that is conducive to mental well-being. A stable condition of an ailing person means that a certain degree of normalcy is achieved. A stable structure means that it is not easily subject to forces that would weaken it and create an imbalance that will jeopardize the strength of the building, and perhaps cause a collapse.

Equality

One definition of balance as it relates to equality is: "to make or be equal to in weight, value, etc.".[1] In mathematics, equality is represented by an equation, a statement of equality between two quantities. The symbol of equality of these two quantities is the equal (=) sign, indicating that the terms on either side of the equation are equal or equivalent. Equality is a concept applied in weighing scales to determine the weight of an object. Once the two sides have equalized, then they are said to be balanced. Weight is determined by the pull of gravity on the mass of an object. Two objects on each side of a scale with the same mass will balance each other.

Equality as a concept has been applied widely in the use of various forms of the weighing scales and measurements in the science of physics. It has also been used as a concept in various spheres of modern life: political, social, and economic. Human rights equality has been an explosive issue in politics. Equality is one of man's highest aspirations—to be treated with equal rights and protection under the law. As a philosophical idea, it has dominated numerous publications, discourses, and discussions. It appears to provide a satisfaction of man's higher need for social recognition and self-esteem.

Well-Being

Well-being is part of the definition of health. It is an integral part of being healthy. Well-being is a state of physical and psychological wellness, not just an absence of disease. It is the individual's perception of their own level of health. The concept of well-being is particularly applied in the field of mental health. The World Health Organization defines mental health as" *"a state of well-being in which every individual realizes his or her own potential, can cope with the normal stresses of life, can work productively and fruitfully, and is able to make a contribution to her or his community"*.[28] This is the positive dimension of mental health as contained in the WHO definition of health.

Internal and external factors can produce an imbalance on a person, thereby affecting the feeling of well-being. Anything that prevents the person from meeting his or her needs—from the physiological to the psychological can lead to an imbalance that in turn affects the person's sense of well-being. The delicate interplay of balance-producing and imbalance-producing factors can affect the person's sense of well-being. Someone who cannot cope with normal stresses of life due to a physical or psychological limitation, cannot realize their own potentials and therefore unable to feel and work productively as a member of society. This affects their self-esteem need, which in turn affects their psychological well-being.

Stresses play an important role in an individual's well-being. As human society becomes more and more complex, the physiological and psychological toll on modern human beings mount. The ability to adapt to these constant changes becomes crucial in the continued survival of man. Contributing to the normal evolutionary processes that human beings undergo over time in response to environmental changes, technological advances have shifted paradigms of existence. Environmental pollutions brought upon our planet from man's own creations and inventions are endangering our very own existence. Societal and cultural changes have made living much more complex. Man is subjected to numerous stresses in everyday life more than ever before in its history. His well-being, health, and survival are compromised unless man himself makes the effort to reverse the process.

———————————•◦•———————————

KEY CONCEPTS:

1. Balance is a universal concept in human existence. The key elements of balance—adaptation, homeostasis, equilibrium, needs and health—are essential to human survival.

2. Balance is the dynamic interplay of all forces that equalize each other within the internal and external environment of the person. Imbalance is the opposite of balance and represents a disruption of any or all the elements of balance.

3. The concept of balance exists in all spheres of human endeavors and variously defined according to the area that it applies.

4. Adaptation is an evolutionary process of physical and psychological changes that all living beings undergo over time in order to survive environmental challenges.

5. Homeostasis is the innate ability of human beings to regulate its internal processes to preserve stability in its internal environment.

6. Equilibrium is the balance of opposing forces influenced by internal and external factors. It also exists in various spheres of human endeavors and variously defined according to the area that it applies.

7. Needs are something that are required for an individual to survive and thrive. Needs are based on a hierarchy, with the most basic for survival at the bottom and the highest psychosocial need at the top.

8. Health is the state of dynamic balance of forces to achieve optimal physical, mental and social well-being and not just the absence of disease or infirmity. Health and balance are intimately connected.

9. Related concepts that are essential in understanding balance in human beings are harmony, symmetry, stability, equality, and well-being.

10. Man is an open system. Balance is maintained within an open system through inputs / stimuli and outputs/behavior to achieve equilibrium. The human being has permeable boundaries that permit the intake, processing of stimuli and outputs in terms of behaviors.

11. A holistic system approach is essential in applying the balance concepts to human beings. It considers not only the individual parts but also the wholeness of the person as it responds to its internal and external environments.

12. Balance is demonstrated through observable, measurable and describable behaviors. These behaviors are balance-seeking to preserve the physiological, physical, and psychosocial integrity of the person.

CHAPTER 1: THE UNIVERSALITY OF BALANCE

REFERENCES

1. Agnes, M. (Ed). 2002. *Webster's New Dictionary and Thesaurus.* Ohio. Wiley Publishing, Inc.

2. Balance definition Free Online Dictionary: http://www.thefreedictionary.com/p/balance. retrieved 4/17/2012.

3. Wong, K. 2012, April. First of our Kind, *Scientific American.*306 (4) 32-39.NY. New York

4. Funk & Wagnalls. 1980. "Man's place in Evolution", in *Atlas of the Human Body.* Chicago, Illinois. Rand McNally & Company.

5. Knierim, J: Neuroscience Online: an Electronic Textbook for the Neurosciences, Cerebellum: Section 3, Chapter 5: http://neuroscience.uth.tmc.edu/s3/chapter 05.html. retrieved 4/06/2012

6. Anderson, D.M. 2005. *Mosby's Medical, Nursing, and Allied Health Dictionary.* (6th ed.) St. Louis. Mosby.

7. Homeostasis : http://en.wikipedia.org/wiki/Homeostasis. retrieved 5/15/2012.

8. Marieb,E and Hoehn, K. 2007. *Human Anatomy & Physiology* (7th ed.) San Francisco, CA. Pearson Benjamin Cummings.

9. Collins, Wm. Sons & Co. Ltd. 2009. *Collins English Dictionary—Complete & Unabridged* (10th ed.). Harper Collins Publishers.

10. Daniels, R. 2002. *Delmar's Guide to Laboratory and Diagnostic Tests.* Albany, New York. Delmar.

11. Libra (Astrology)—Wikipedia: http//en.wikipedia.org/wiki/Libra_(astrology). Retrieved 3/23/2011

12. Petruso, Karl M. Early Weights and Weighing in Egypt and the Indus Valley, M Bulletin (Boston Museum of Fine Arts,), Vol. 79, (1981) pp. 44-51(http://www.jstor.org/stable/4171634) *retrieved 3/23/12.*

13. Sanders, L. A. (rev. 1960). Short history of weighing. Birmingham, England, W. & T. Avery, (http://www.averyweigh-tronix.com/download.aspx?did=6249. Retrieved 3/25/2011

14. Spector, R. 2009. *Cultural Diversity in Health and Illness.* (7th ed.) Upper Saddle River, New Jersey. Pearson Prentice Hall.

15. Venes, D. (Ed.) 2005. *Taber's Cyclopedic Medical Dictionary.* Philadelphia. F.A. Davis

16. Maslow's hierarchy of needs: http://en.wikipedia.org/wiki/Maslow's hierarchy of needs. retrieved 05/22/2012.

17. Christensen, B.L. and Kockrow, E.O.2006. *Foundations of Nursing* (5th ed.) Philadelphia. Mosby Elsevier.

18. Maslow, A. 1970. *Motivation and Personality* (2nd ed.) New York. Harper & Row.

19. Giger, J.N. and Davidhizar, R.E. 1995. *Transcultural Nursing Assessment and Intervention*, (2nd ed.). St. Louis, MO. Mosby-Year Book, Inc.

20. Preamble to the Constitution of the World Health Organization as adopted by the International Health Conference, New York, 19-22 June, 1946; signed on 22 July 1946 by representatives of 61 States (Official Records of the World Health Organization, no. 2, p.100) and entered into force on 7 April 1948.

21. Heylighen, F. and Joslyn C. 1992. "What is Systems Theory". Principia Cybernetica: http://pespmc1.vub.ac.be/SYSTHEOR.html. retrieved 4/14/2012.

22. Hutchison, E.D.2003. *Dimensions of Human Behavior: Person and Environment* (2nd ed.) Thousand Oaks. Sage.

23. Systems Theory/Open/Closed System: http://en.wikibooks.org/wiki/Systems_Theory/Open/Closed_System_Structure&oldid. retrieved 4/14/2012.

24. Systems Theory/Holism: http://enwikibooks.org/wiki/Systems_Theory/Holism.retrieved 4/14/2012.

25. Mason, B. Taoist Principles: http://www.taoism.net/articles/mason/principl.html. retrieved 4/3/2012.

26. Kauffman III, W.J. and Freedman, R.A.1994. *Gravitation and the Motions of the Planets and Universe* (5th ed.) New York. Freeman and Company.

27. Equilibrium: http://en.wikipedia.org/wiki/Equilibrium. retrieved 4/3/2012

28. WHO/Mental Health: a state of well-being: http://.www.who.int/features/factfiles/mental_health/en/index.html. retrieved3/24/2012

TABLE 1.1: Balance Concepts in the Sciences, Arts, and Other Fields

<u>Equilibrium</u> Physics Chemistry Anatomy Geometry	<u>Homeostasis</u> Physiology Biological Science Medicine
<u>Symmetry</u> Architecture Painting Design	<u>Harmony</u> Music Psychology Culture Religion /Spirituality
<u>Equality</u> Mathematics Economics Accounting Sociology	<u>Balance of Nature</u> Ecology Environmental Science Geology

<u>Holistic</u>

Nursing
Wellness
Health Sciences
Alternative Medicine

DIAGRAM 1.3 Conceptual Representation: Balance. Five Elements, and influencing factors in Survival

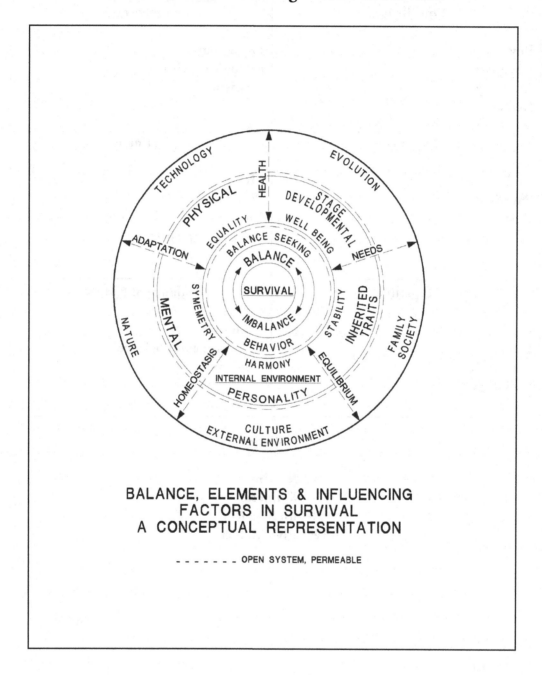

BALANCE, ELEMENTS & INFLUENCING
FACTORS IN SURVIVAL
A CONCEPTUAL REPRESENTATION

- - - - - - - OPEN SYSTEM, PERMEABLE

DIAGRAM 1.4 BALANCE CONCEPT MAP

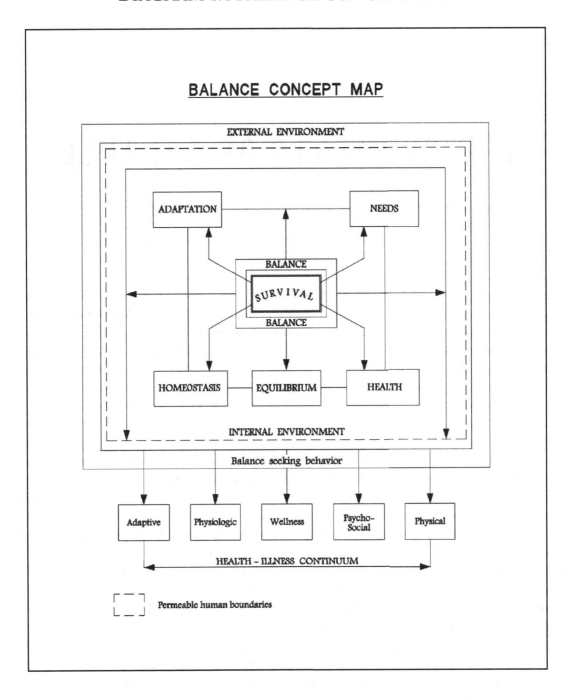

BALANCE CONCEPT MAP

EXTERNAL ENVIRONMENT

ADAPTATION

NEEDS

BALANCE

SURVIVAL

BALANCE

HOMEOSTASIS

EQUILIBRIUM

HEALTH

INTERNAL ENVIRONMENT

Balance seeking behavior

Adaptive

Physiologic

Wellness

Psycho-Social

Physical

HEALTH – ILLNESS CONTINUUM

⌐ ¬
⌊ ⌋ Permeable human boundaries

Chapter 2

ENVIRONMENTS OF BALANCE

"Nothing endures but change."
—Heraclitus (540 BC-480 BC)

This chapter discusses further the elements in the internal and external environment of the human being that affect balance, and ultimately his survival in this planet. First, it is important to look at the concept of the human being as an open system. By doing so, it becomes logical to consider the environments, internal and external, that affect the individual. Next, the internal and external factors that affect all of us need to be discussed to give a holistic view of the human being. Equilibrium as an underlying force that balances the elements in the internal environment and the elements in the external environment have to be considered.

The concept of change as part of the dynamic interplay of internal and external forces or stimuli and the exchange of information, energy and matter across the open system have to be major considerations. It is just as important to consider change as a constant in an evolving world. Nothing stays the same in man's constant and dynamic interaction with the environment. While the concept of change does not seem to be consistent with balance, it actually is part of human existence. The dynamic interrelationship between man and his internal and external environment suggests a constant adjustment to the influx of stimuli in order to maintain balance. As the planet moves in its axis and around the solar system, all of earth's inhabitants are also affected by this movement. Balancing forces have to be at play to maintain equilibrium. The human engine of cellular metabolism is constantly humming with activity to keep the body alive without our control. Blood circulates in the veins as long as the heart beats. And every beat of that heart is separate from the one before it and the one after it. Anything can interrupt this rhythm. Realities change from one moment to the next. Since moments are fragments of time, and "time flows in a single direction, from past to future",[1] the state we were in a moment ago is not the same state we are in present time, and in the future.

HUMAN BEING AS AN OPEN SYSTEM

An open system is one which continuously interacts with the environment. This interaction can take the form of information, energy, or material that moves in and out the system's boundary. It is based on the Systems theory originally proposed in the 1940s by biologist Ludwig von Bertalanffy who emphasized that real systems are open to, and interact with their environments and in the process can acquire new properties resulting in a continual evolution.[2] Rather than focusing on independent parts, the systems theory also focuses on the interrelationship between the parts that make up the whole entity. The Systems theory has gained wide application in various fields such as information technology, sociology, physics, biology, engineering, ecology, computing, nursing, and studies of human behavior.

The view that the human being is an open system is compatible with what is generally known about human nature: that man constantly interacts with his environment. We possess biologic boundaries and structures in our bodies that make us permeable to outside stimuli, process the stimuli so that we can adjust quickly and adapt if necessary, and deliver outputs that are manifested internally or externally. Because of this permeability, the environment can affect the human system, and it can also affect the environment. This enables the human being to adapt to changes, sustain its growth and increase its probability of survival. In studying the structures, functions and processes of the human body, one cannot escape the wonder of its immense complexity, and yet, it has managed to function as a well-coordinated body, capable of yet even greater feats of the intellect. Understanding those forces that keep the body in balance within itself and the world around him helps in understanding man's continued quest for survival.

The human system only serves as a framework for the intake and output of stimuli from the environment. It has an internal environment biologically hardwired so that it could deal with influences that are both beneficial and dangerous to the human system. The internal regulatory mechanism called *homeostasis* functions round the clock, asleep or awake, to keep the fire of life burning. Higher centers in the brain control these mechanisms through chemical and hormonal actions released by various organs under the control of this "command center" called the brain.It also has built in defense mechanisms that protect the human body from invasion of foreign substances that could pose a threat to its health, well-being and survival.

The external environment is an entirely different entity that human beings have to manipulate in order to meet their needs—from the basic physiologic level to higher forms of psychosocial needs, using Maslow's framework of the hierarchy of needs. The external environment is replete with stimuli and provides a barrage of input—physical and psychological. Human beings have to process and selectively respond to these stimuli so as not to overwhelm the system. Since these inputs are different from one individual to another, their behavioral responses could be quite different. How these inputs are also processed psychologically by each individual depend on a number of influencing factors such as mental and physical health, personality, inherited traits, developmental stage, cultural background, gender, and past experiences. Herein lie the individuality and diversity of human beings. External environmental factors include stress, culture, roles in society, environmental elements, technology, not to mention forces that affect our planet and the universe. However, the secrets to the mind-body-environment connection have yet to be fully unlocked by science.

EQUILIBRIUM IN THE INTERNAL AND EXTERNAL ENVIRONMENTS

Equilibrium is generally defined as a state of balance between opposing forces. It is also defined as "the condition of a system in which competing influences are balanced". The term "equilibrium" have been used along with related terms in traditional science like stability, order, and uniformity. These concepts are generally used synonymously in the definition of balance. The concept of equilibrium applied in the fields of physics, chemistry, and biology continues to be the subject of study and research. Scientific thoughts also consider that changes happen when factors are introduced in the system that disturb this equilibrium. It appears that although a state of disequilibrium occurs, balancing forces manage to get the system back to a state of stability through various processes.

As had been mentioned earlier, the innate sense of balance already exists in human beings as part of the evolutionary process of human development. The sense of balance is regulated by the brain in the cerebellum. Sensory input from the outside environment is obtained by the vestibular system, the sensory apparatus of the inner ear. The information fed by the vestibular system is processed in the cerebellum which makes adjustments in order to maintain balance. As a two-legged animal, man has to have a fine-tuned sense of physical balance in order to walk with stability and adjusts to shifts in body position and changes in the load on the body. [3]

The opposite of equilibrium is disequilibrium or a state of *imbalance.* Whenever elements exist that change the dynamics of the equilibrium, it results in a state of disequilibrium. This state places the system in an unstable state or a disorder, if you will, of the organized state of affairs in a state of equilibrium. In order for the system to go back to a state of relative equilibrium and balance, opposing forces have to neutralize each other. This state or degree of disorder or chaos is called **entropy**.[4,1] This concept of equilibrium/disequilibrium will be important later on in the discussion of wellness and illness.

THE INTERNAL ENVIRONMENT: LIFE SUPPORT SYSTEMS, HOMEOSTASIS, STRESS RESPONSE, DEFENSE MECHANISMS, AND IMMUNITY

Life support systems

What inside the body holds the key to life itself? If balance is the foundation of survival, what is the key that turns life on and off? This is as much a scientific question as a philosophical one. The brain appears to be the anatomic structure that supports the answer. As the central command of all input and output of energy to and from the human body, the brain exerts overall control of life's processes. The functions of the brain appeared to have developed according to its importance to survival.[3] The functions vital to survival are respirations, heart beat, and circulation. Oxygen is the element needed by the cells to stay alive. This element needs to be taken in from the external environment through an open airway and circulated throughout the body by the human pump, the heart. The vital center that controls these functions is in the part of the brain that developed first in the evolutionary process—the brain stem.

Situated deep inside the brain stem is a lattice-work of cells called the **reticular formation** within which lies the basic life-support systems. It also controls level of consciousness. The cells controlling consciousness form a chain that travels through the center of the brain stem to the midbrain and spreads to the upper layers of the brain, the cerebral cortex, where information is processed. Whether conscious or not, the vital centers in the reticular formation in the brain stem continues to perform its primeval duty: to support life automatically through processes emanating from the reticular formation.

Be that as it may, the control functions of the reticular formation to support life cannot be executed without those other vital organs of respirations, heartbeat, and circulation of the vital elements of life—oxygen and fluids. The brain itself needs to preserve its cellular integrity to function. Advances in medical science have developed mechanical life support systems for human beings without the capability to breathe, circulate oxygen via the blood stream, and maintain heartbeat. These organs have to work collaboratively with each other in order to maintain the balance of vital elements needed for survival. Without cellular integrity, and balance of elements essential to cellular life, the key to survival will be turned off.

Homeostasis: internal physiologic balance

Another important concept related to the principle of balance in man and other biologic beings is homeostasis. It is a physiologic process which refers to the ability or tendency of an organism or cell to maintain internal equilibrium through automatic regulation of physiologic processes. As mentioned previously, the ability or tendency of an organism or cell to maintain internal equilibrium by adjusting its physiological processes. It is also broadly defined as an equilibrium among psychological, physiological, sociocultural, intellectual, and spiritual needs.[5] This state of equilibrium in the internal environment is naturally maintained by adaptive responses that promote health and survival. The organ primarily responsible for regulating homeostasis is the hypothalamus.

When a human being experiences a stimulus whether internal or external, this signal is sent to that center in the brain that processes this information and stimulates the individual to respond. The stimuli can be interpreted by the body as stress. It is defined in many other ways as: 1) a nonspecific physiological response to a stimulus which could be perceived by the person as pleasant or unpleasant experience that evokes a change; 2) a change in the environment perceived as threatening to one's equilibrium; 3) related to a continued wear and tear on the body over time; and 4) psychological stress from internal or environmental events as interpreted by the person.[6] This creates an imbalance or a physiologic change in the body that requires for it to return to its former natural state of balance. *The natural tendency of human beings is to correct the imbalance.* The internal physiologic response involves processes set into motion by the body to correct the imbalance regardless of external conditions. These physiologic responses involve an adaptive response to return the body to its former state of balance for its survival.

Fluids and electrolyte balance is an example of how the body maintains homeostasis.[6,7,8] Water balance is maintained via a complex process regulated by the hypothalamus in the brain interacting with the pituitary gland and the kidneys to release hormones that regulate the absorption or excretion of water. Thru internal mechanisms, the body moves fluids in and out of its various compartments to achieve homeostasis. These processes utilize principles of physics to move fluids and electrolytes through intracellular and extracellular compartments. All these happen as part of the natural process of homeostasis and not regulated by conscious thought.

There are two major fluid compartments of the body. These fluids need to be balanced in order to maintain homeostasis. These are: 1) intracellular fluid (ICF) located within the cells and constitutes approximately 40% of body weight, and 2) extracellular fluid (ECF) located outside of the cell. Electrolytes are substances present in the body whose molecules are composed of two electrically charged particles called **ions** that are either positively charged or negatively charged. Cations are positively charged particles, and anions are negatively charged. Cations and anions combine or dissociate according to the chemical processes involved.

Principles of chemistry and physics are used in understanding the movements of ions and molecules. Under normal conditions, the body maintains this balance of fluids between the intracellular and the extracellular compartments to maintain homeostasis. Fluid and electrolyte imbalance is a condition that needs to be corrected to achieve homeostasis once again. Conditions such as dehydration or edema occur in individuals with illness and disrupt the normal homeostatic mechanism.

The primary organs for regulating fluid and electrolyte balance are the kidneys through adjustments in the fluid intake and output. Urine formation starts in the kidneys where a very complex process of filtration, reabsorption, secretion and excretion of water, electrolytes and waste products of metabolism occur. Other organs of the body also participate in regulation of fluids and of internal homeostasis through interrelated and highly integrated processes involving various systems such as the cardiovascular system, gastrointestinal system, the respiratory system, and the integumentary system. The mechanisms controlling fluids and electrolytes in the body are governed by principles of physics and chemistry such as diffusion, filtration, osmosis, and hydrostatic pressure.

Diffusion is the movement of molecules from an area of high concentration to an area of lower concentration. When the concentrations of each side are equal, the net movement from one area to another ceases. This state of stability achieved with the diffusion of molecules to equalize concentration is a balanced state. Diffusion not only occurs in liquids but also in gases and solids. When a membrane separates these two areas, diffusion can only occur if that membrane is **permeable**. Simple diffusion does not require application of external energy e.g., heat. The process of diffusion facilitates the movement of fluid from the intracellular fluid to the extracellular compartment, and vice versa, depending on the concentration of molecules on each side. The concept of permeability is also applied in systems, such as the human being when interacting with the external environment. This permeability allows the body to receive outside stimuli to be processed internally and manifested outwardly in behaviors.

Osmosis is the movement of water between two compartments separated by a semipermeable membrane, a membrane permeable to water but not to a solute. The concept of balance also applies in the principle of osmosis in chemistry. Water moves through the membrane from an area of low solute concentration to an area of high solute concentration. In other words, water moves from a more concentrated to a less concentrated area. When the differences in concentration between two sides disappear, or when hydrostatic pressure builds up that is sufficient to oppose any further movement of the water, the solution achieves a stable state (no movement occurs). In the human body, the glomerulus is a semi-permeable membrane that allows fluid to pass through in the process of urine formation.

Hydrostatic pressure is the pressure exerted by a fluid at equilibrium in proportion to the amount of fluid in a column or container influenced by the force of gravity. It also depends on the density of the fluid. In the human body, hydrostatic pressure present in the glomerular capillaries is generated by the force of the contraction of the heart through the vascular tree. The causes a certain amount of blood to be filtered across the semipermeable membranes in the glomerulus where the filtered fluid passes through the different tubules and ducts of the kidneys. The final product of this highly complex process is the urine. Perhaps unknown to many people, the urine is a product that represents the exquisite balance that the body maintains internally to keep on surviving and thriving through well-functioning internal systems.

Physiologic stress response

A certain amount of stress is necessary for survival as it enables the body to mobilize its resources continuously and adapt to its environmental demands. The stimuli that evokes a need to adapt is called a **stressor.** The nature of the stressor can be classified as physiologic, physical, and psychosocial. It is related to the level of need in Maslow's hierarchy. Physiologic stress conditions such as oxygen deprivation, fluid and electrolyte imbalances, and dehydration are directly related to basic physiologic needs. Physical stressors are anything perceived by the individual as threatening to that person's sense of safety and security, such as accidents and natural and man-made disasters. When confronted with an immediate physical danger that could endanger his life, the fight or flight behavioral response is triggered as a survival mechanism. Psychosocial stressors are those that are more directly related to belonging and esteem needs. If especially prolonged, these stressors require adaptive coping mechanisms.

The threat could be real or imagined as interpreted by the person and requires adaptive behavior for the individual dealing with stress over time. The goal of adaptive behavior is to achieve homeostasis, which is the equilibrium between physiological, psychological, socio-cultural, intellectual, and spiritual needs. Disequilibrium results when stress overwhelms the body's normal coping resources, which could be physiologic and psychologic.[7,8] The physiologic response to stress is the "fight or flight" reaction originally proposed by Walter Cannon over 60 years ago and expanded by Hans Selye in his **General Adaptation Syndrome (GAS)**.Hans Selye described this as the *General Adaptation Response (GAS)*.[5,6,8] In order for the body to adjust effectively, the body undergoes several stages before it gradually returns to normal equilibrium and stability. The three stages of GAS are: 1) alarm reaction, 2) stage of resistance, and 3) stage of exhaustion. Internal reaction is manifested through the activation of the three stages of the GAS and fairly universal.

Initially, the alarm stage that starts in the hypothalamus, spreads to the posterior pituitary, the anterior pituitary, the sympathetic nervous system and the medulla, triggering the "fight or flight" response. This creates a disturbance or disruption of the normal processes of the internal environment. During the resistance stage, the body starts to go back to stability, with hormonal levels returning to normal, parasympathetic nervous system activities take over, and the individual begins to adapt to the stressors. Recovery then returns the person to equilibrium. Prolonged state of stress or inability of the individual to stabilize the internal environment through effective coping can push the individual to the exhaustion stage. The stress response at this stage is manifested by continued or increased physiologic response as in the alarm stage, decreased energy levels and decreased physiological adaptation. Examples of these changes are those that involve the heart, blood vessels, lungs, adrenal medulla, liver and the gastrointestinal systems. This creates imbalances that, if not returned to normal equilibrium will pose a threat to the individual's health and well-being. Progressive continued imbalances will ultimately lead to death unless reversed. The intimate relationship between the internal and external environments can be well appreciated in stress situations.

Prolonged psychological stress that exceeds a person's ability to return to psychological equilibrium through normal coping strategies can cause physical and psychological disorders. Stress-related disease and conditions include coronary heart disease, hypertension, stroke, stomach ulcers, diabetes, ulcerative colitis, depression, and insomnia. The effects of stress on the immune system is now well-recognized.

Defense mechanisms and immunity

The human body also has built-in defense and repair mechanisms within the internal environment to protect is integrity from invasion of foreign substances such as bacteria, viruses, parasites, and injury.[3,8] Despite constant attacks from these biological, as well as damaging physical elements from the external environment, the human body has managed to adapt and survive through a range of defense mechanisms and repair systems. Scientific understanding of these natural defenses has contributed to advances in modern medicine and contributed to man's longevity and health at this point in time in its history. Breakdown of these natural defenses interrupt the normal functioning of human systems. This causes an imbalance in the form of disease processes, inflammation or injury. If this imbalance is allowed to continue without intervention or natural recovery, the body would eventually be unable to maintain balance between the invading forces and its defense mechanisms, thereby leading to its demise.

The ability of the body to ward off infections and protect itself from noxious elements requires a constant balancing act between its natural defenses and the injurious effects of the invaders. Worse, there are many organisms that are permanent residents in our bodies. However, not all microorganism cause harm to the body under normal circumstances. It is when the body's defenses weaken or break down that these microorganisms proliferate and overrun the body.

The intricate layers of defense of the body start with the skin which is the first line of defense and a major barrier of the body. The skin, with its tough, flexible, self-repairing and water-proof qualities, protect the internal layers and organs of the body. The brain, the body's most important software, is protected by a bony structure called the skull. The mucous membranes of the alimentary and respiratory tracts also have protective filter mechanisms and chemicals that further act as a barrier to try to ward off the foreign substances. The main object of the primary line of defense is to keep organisms from getting into the blood stream and carried to different parts of the body where they can lodge and thrive.

If organisms do succeed in penetrating the first line of defense and enter the blood stream, they are attacked by cells produced in the reticuloendothelial system, neutralized and disposed of. Starting with the white blood cells, these and other white cells that reside in the lymph nodes, spleen, liver, bone marrow, and lungs in the reticuloendothelial system, surround and engulf these organisms and particles. The lymphatic system, the fluid that surrounds the body's cells, has lymph nodes that act as filters through the white cells that ingest these microorganisms, thus preventing them from gaining access to the blood stream. Should the lymphatic system fail to filter out these organisms, there is another line of defense within the cells of the spleen, liver and bone marrow.

Furthermore, the immune system provides an important back-up protection via a major complex chemical system which deactivates some organisms and neutralizes the toxins they produce. This system, called the immune response, consists of white blood cells and lymphocytes that are always circulating in the blood stream, like marching sentries guarding the castle. The presence of an organism like bacteria activates the lymphocytes and induces an immune response. Any substance that causes an immune response is called an antigen. T-lymphocytes, a type of lymphocyte, becomes active when it gets in contact with an antigen. This contact with the invading microorganism produces a substance called **antibody**. The antibody in turn breaks down the external membrane of the organism, thereby destroying it. Antibodies are capable of destroying bacteria, viruses and other microorganisms, thus protecting the body from these disease-causing elements.

EXTERNAL/EXTRINSIC ENVIRONMENTS: PHYSICAL AND PSYCHOSOCIAL FACTORS

Leaving the wondrous mechanisms inside the human body, we then look at stimuli in the external environment which also affect the internal balance of the human beings. These stimuli outside of the human body are processed by the human being via sensory input through its sensory organs: the eyes, ears, nose, and skin relayed to the brain for processing via the sensory pathways. Additionally, the human being also has the capacity to involve his higher thinking abilities to perceive and evaluate the stimuli through interaction with the outside environment. This determines how the individual responds to the external stimuli which could be a situation, an inanimate (non-living) object, or animate (living) object. This response could be conscious and deliberate, or reflexive, and vary from individual to individual depending on numerous factors both innate and outwardly determined. Such factors as personality, previous experiences, health, cultural background and beliefs, family and societal influences, socio-economic conditions, and environmental factors all play a part in determining individual responses. These reflect the individual's attempt to deal with the stressful stimuli and return the body to its normal and stable state.

Presuming that the vital elements that critically support life, such as oxygen and nitrogen, are available and elements that do not support life, such as carbon dioxide and other poisonous gases, are not present in sufficient amounts to be harmful to life, other basic elements from the environment become critically important. Environmental factors such as heat, cold, climate, weather, pollution, wind, rain, air movements, snow, earthquakes, ferocious animals, etc. are common denominators to human existence, depending on their geographical locations in the planet. To respond to the basic need of safety, man has to utilize resources within his capabilities to protect himself from the harmful elements in nature. Through the use of his well-developed brain, man had been able to negotiate through the ages with those external elements that threatened his survival. By having the natural instinct to seek other human beings and form social groups, man had been able to survive even further. As generally accepted by biologists, man is biologically engineered to adapt. Culture is one of the results of having a highly adaptive mind.[9] It appears that the development of culture has a protective function in human development.

Physical: The elements of nature

The physical environment outside the body is a major determinant of survival. In the course of human history, catastrophic events of nature, such as earthquakes, volcanic eruptions, tornadoes, hurricanes, tsunamis, floods, etc. have decimated populations of the earth's inhabitants. Climatic changes bringing about drought, famine, and extreme temperatures have influenced movements of people in search of food, water, and shelter to ensure their survival. Archaeologists and geneticists have theorized that the migratory movements of early humans followed the coastal route as a sort of "prehistoric superhighway".[9] which facilitated rapid migration and proximity to sources of food from the sea. What prompted them to travel long distances and brave the harsh environments in search of food and water, is what I suspect as responding to their basic need for survival. This behavior does not seem different in motivation than driving to the grocery store to buy food. Food is a basic human need that has remained constant in human beings.

The importance of the environment in maintaining health has been recognized even from the early days of nursing. Florence Nightingale recognized the influence of environmental factors on health and illness. In her "Notes on Nursing", she wrote in detail her ideas on environmental cleanliness, water supply, sanitation, sunlight, ventilation and warming, on caring for patients. She also recognized the effect of ". . . . climates of the earth that are meant to be made habitable for man . . . ."[10] This environmental component of the care of patients has been a lasting concept utilized in health care and nursing until the present time.

Psychosocial factors: Stressors

Neuman defines stressors as disruptive forces operating within or on any system. [10,7] Stressors are environmental demands that impinge on the person. These demands could be in terms of situations, relationships, or events that are significant enough to the person. The manner that people interpret the influence of stressors on themselves depends on their appraisal of the situation. Stress is universal to all human beings and is necessary for survival. It affects every person regardless of age, gender, race, economic condition, educational level or culture. How the person deals with the stressors depend on the individual's coping abilities. Coping is the person's effort to manage psychological stress. [12,7]. It is the person's adaptive behavioral response to achieve mental and emotional equilibrium to maintain balance.

It is notable to point out the role of adaptation in the process of adjusting to stressors. As discussed in earlier chapter, it is one of the critical elements of the concept of balance. Adaptation in this context is an ongoing process by which individuals make adjustments physically, physiologically, psychologically, intellectually, and socio-culturally in response to stressors in order to achieve homeostasis. A broader meaning of homeostasis is applied to the steady state in all dimensions of life. It is also called equilibrium.

Response to stressors is affected by many factors that depend on the person's appraisal of the following: the intensity of the stressor, the scope, duration, number and nature of other stressors, and predictability. Psychological stress differ in each person and produces different behavioral reactions. The characteristics of the individual also influence the stress response and these are: level of personal control, availability of social supports, feelings of competence, and cognitive appraisal.[7] Maturational factors also play a role in how people cope with stressors. The person's ability to exercise critical thinking and logical process to assess the stressor, as well as the ability to use problem-solving techniques, will also determine the kind of behavior the person will exhibit to respond to a situation. This involves higher level of thought processing that reflects the level of behavior the person has achieved in the behavioral pyramid (see Behavioral pyramid diagram). This level is the intellectual/rational realm of human behavior.

There are two types of stress according to the general outcome:[7] one is called **eustress**, a type that produces a positive outcome, such as a swimmer who experiences stress while preparing for a competition. This challenges him to be physically fit for the competition and goes on to win it. On the other hand, one that results in a negative or ineffective response is called **distress.** When a person is unable to cope with stressors, a **crisis** results. This is a state of disequilibrium that is time-limited. With appropriate intervention and support, the crisis can be resolved. There are three basic factors that help the individual resolve a crisis and these are: the person's perception, coping mechanisms, and situational support.[5] If one, or all, of these factors is missing, the individual feels mentally out of balance. Resolution of the crisis allows the individual to restore a sense of equilibrium and balance.

Besides the physical elements, the stressors experienced by the individual from the external environment come from psychosocial factors. Social relationships with family, co-workers, and others in society pose constant challenges and stresses in the modern world. Additionally, rapidly advancing technology changes the dynamics of these relationships. These factors are destabilizing to individuals unless they find a way to adapt to them through positive coping mechanisms. Change, a constant in human existence, seems to happen even faster. And those unable to cope with the changing times could find these unsettling and destabilizing to the equilibrium.

In the need to find balance, modern individuals adopt balance-seeking behaviors, those behaviors that enable human beings to maintain a steady state of equilibrium. Whether the impetus comes from within the internal environment or from the external environment, balancing behaviors tend to seek a level of equilibrium physiologically, physically, and psychosocially. It enables individuals to respond to, and adapt to changes and factors producing imbalances. Adaptation is the process that has enabled humans to survive and thrive throughout the ages. It is also part of cultural norms that had evolved over time with the balancing messages from a well-developed brain. The protective function of culture plays a major role in providing a sense of balance that all humans seek. The predictability of cultural elements make it a source of safety and stability for individuals. The influence of culture will be discussed in another section.

BALANCE OF OPPOSING FORCES

The environment of human beings is replete with opposing forces that need to be maintained in a balance so that one force does not dominate another. In the center of the earth is the gravitational pull that enables beings on the surface of the planet to stay in place and not fly off to space. Gravity is the force that is always present in the environment and is the same force that attracts all objects to each other. The law that governs this is Newton's law of Universal Gravitation.[13,14] The size of this force depends on two factors: the mass of the objects and the distance between them. Forces that are opposite in direction and equal in size are called balanced forces. Opposing forces that are not equal create an imbalance. As in a weighing scale, if one side is greater than the other and not counterbalanced, the scale will tip in the direction of the greater force.

This is perhaps how the concept of opposites sprang from. Opposites actually are part of the continuum of wholeness: opposing forces tend to equalize each other to find a point of equilibrium where stability is found. Striving for wholeness and balance seems to be an innate need common to all human beings since they started becoming the intelligent beings that they are, up to the present time. This point of stability is also a zone where the person can find the highest point of well-being, equilibrium and harmony.

Opposing forces in the environment and in nature may have always existed since the beginning of time. For thousands of years, mankind have delved into the mysteries of opposites, opposing forces they have observed in nature and human behavior. These forces have affected human beings in a variety of ways that are not necessary felt or seen. These forces of nature exerting its effects on our bodies are probably more intuitively felt and responded to in many ways over the ages. For instance, opposing forces can find its way in peoples' way of life, health, behavior, science, technologies, creativity, and spirituality. Balancing these opposing forces have been part of human existence. It is the foundation of some religious and healthcare care beliefs. Some examples of these forces found in human behaviors, social systems and bio-physical systems are: equilibrium vs. disequilibrium, harmony vs. disharmony, symmetry vs. asymmetry, equality vs. inequality; Yin and Yang; elements of nature such as fire and water, heat and cold, abundance vs. deprivation, etc.

The concept of opposites seems to dominate human existence. At the primal level, opposites define human existence. The heat of the sun, the source of all energy on earth, is balanced with the coldness of night; the north pole vs. the south pole; for every sunrise, there is a sunset; for every storm there is calm; every ebb of the ocean tide has a flow, a beginning of life and end of life, as birth and death. In human emotions, there are high's and low's, sadness and happiness, satisfaction and dissatisfaction, joy and sorrow, pain and pleasure, love and hate. Opposites are two ends of the continuum acting to balance each other's influences. The dualistic nature[15] of opposites are found in many aspects of our existence and our physical bodies: female vs. male; left and right sides; our left brain and right brain, health and illness; The whole range of our physical and psychological existence happen within the continuum of opposites and found its way into our cultural practices and beliefs.

It is in finding the center of the two extreme poles of opposing forces where the most harmony and balance can be found. This is where human beings find their best place in the universe.

KEY CONCEPTS

1. Understanding the internal and external environments that support survival provides a holistic approach to the concept of balance.
2. The influences of homeostasis and equilibrium applied to human systems utilize scientific principles in physics and chemistry.
3. Disturbances of homeostasis and equilibrium produce disequilibrium, imbalance and decreased well-being.
4. Human beings are open systems that continuously receive inputs, process these inputs, and deliver outputs through permeable boundaries to regulate itself for survival.
5. The internal environments of basic life support, homeostasis, physiologic stress response, defense mechanisms, and immunity support continued survival and growth.
6. The internal homeostatic processes of diffusion, osmosis, and hydrostatic pressure are governed by scientific principles of chemistry and physics.
7. Physiologic stress responses, described by Hans Selye as "General Adaptation Syndrome" (GAS), create a change in the internal environment in response to stress, and create an imbalance. The three stages of GAS enable the person to flee from or fight the perceived threat, then return to equilibrium when the threat is gone.
8. Psychologic sources of stress come from the external environment perceived by the individual as positive or negative. Coping abilities to stressors enable individuals to adapt to constant stress.
9. Balance-seeking behaviors enable human beings to maintain a steady state of equilibrium.
10. Culture developed over time as part of balance-seeking behavior governed by messages from the brain has a protective function to support man's striving for survival.
11. Opposing forces are found in all aspects of the physical and psychological characteristics of human beings and part of the dualistic nature of existence. These forces are opposite poles in the continuum acting to balance each other's influences. The center of the two opposing poles is where equilibrium, harmony, and balance can be found.

CHAPTER 2: Environments of Balance

REFERENCES

1. Prigogine, Ilya. 1984. "Irreversibility—The Entropy Barrier". In *Order Out of Chaos*. New York. Bantam Books. 277-278.

2. Heylighten, F. and Joslyn C.1992 What is Systems Theory? Prepared for the Cambridge Dictionary of Philosophy. Cambridge University Press. Http://pespmc1.vub.ac.be/SYSTHEOR.HTML.retrieved 4/14/2012.

3. Funk & Wagnalls. 1980. *Atlas of the Human Body*. Chicago & NewYork. Rand McNally & Company.

4. Venes, D.(Ed). 2005.*Taber's Cyclopedic Medical Dictionary* (20th ed.) Philadelphia. F.A. Davis Company.

5. Daniels,R., Grendell, R.N., Wilkins, F.R. 2010. *Nursing Fundamentals: Caring & Clinical Decision-Making* (2nd ed.) Clifton Park, New York. Delmar Cengage.

6. Lewis, S.L., et.al. 2007. *Medical-Surgical Nursing: Assessment and Management of Clinical Problems (7th ed.)* St. Louis, MO.Mosby.

7. Potter, P.A. & Perry, A.G. 2005. *Fundamentals of Nursing (6th ed.)*. St. Louis, MO. Mosby.

8. Huether, S.E. and McCance, K.L. 2008. *Understanding Pathophysiology (4th ed.)* St. Louis, MO. Mosby.

9. Wells, S. 2002. *The Journey of Man: A Genetic Odyssey*. New Jersey. Princeton University Press.

10. Nightingale, F.1860. *Notes on Nursing*. Republished in New York (1969). Dover publications. (from replication of the first American edition in 1860 by D. Appleton and Company).

11. Neuman, B. 1995. *The Neuman Systems Model (3rd ed.)* Stamford, Conn. Appleton & Lange.

12. Lazarus, R. 1999. *Stress and Emotion: A New Synthesis*. New York. Springer.

13. Hurd, D., et.al. 1988. *Physical Science*. Englewood Cliffs, New Jersey. Prentice-Hall, Inc.

14. Kauffmann III, W. & Freedman, R. 1999. *Universe* (5th ed.). New York. W.H. Freeman and Company.

15. Opposites and Balance. http://www.universal-mind.org//Opposites_and balance.html. retrieved 7/01/2012.

LIST OF STRESSORS

1. **PHYSIOLOGIC** (directly related to basic physiologic needs)

   Pain
   Infection and inflammation
   Cancers
   Diseases and disorders
   Traumatic injuries
   Surgery
   Oxygenation dysfunction
   Fluid and Electrolyte imbalances
   Dehydration
   Malnutrition
   Bleeding/hematologic conditions
   Immune Disorders
   Elimination dysfunctions
   Pregnancy
   Neurologic disorders
   Adverse effects of medications
   Addiction

2. **PHYSICAL** (directly related to safety and security)
   Extreme temperatures
   Environmental pollution
   Climate changes—drought, snow, rain
   Natural disasters—storm, hurricane, tornado, earthquake, famine, flood,
   Man—made disasters—fire, bombs. chemical spills, terrorism, war,
   Homelessness
   Accidents and trauma
   Immobility
   Allergies

3. **PSYCHOSOCIAL** (indirectly related to safety and security; directly related to belonging and esteem)

   Loss of loved one—death, divorce, separation
   Low self-concept or body image
   Dysfunctional family

Sexual dysfunction
Conflict—interpersonal, organizational
Poverty
Powerlessness
Discrimination and inequality
Care giving strain
Parenting
Care-giving
Rape
Hopelessness
Immaturity
Relocation
Domestic violence
Loss of job or source of income
Rejection
Neglect
Aging
Ethical dilemmas
Role expectations
Cultural conflicts and expectations
Fears and phobias
Sexual dysfunction

DIAGRAM 2.1 MAN AS AN OPEN SYSTEM

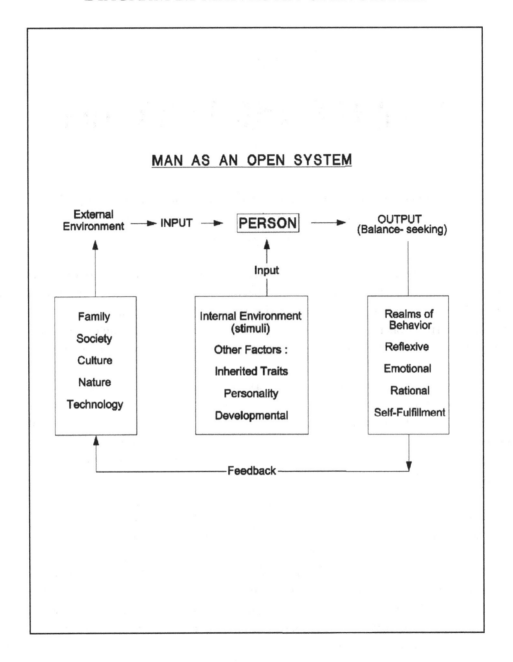

Chapter 3

BALANCE AND BEHAVIOR

"Our humanity rests upon a series of learned behaviors, woven together into patterns that are infinitely fragile and never directly inherited".
—*Margaret Mead*

Behavior is a characteristic of all living human beings. It is also a commonality among other species in the animal kingdom. The difference between behavior of animals and human beings is the use of mental processing and deliberative thought uniquely characteristic of intelligent human beings. The great mystery of human behavior at this time, is the question of how the human brain processes information received and reacts to it in a reasonable and appropriate manner through behaviors. It is a known fact that there are many factors that affect behavior, and differences exist in their exterior characteristics, such as color, features, posture, height, weight, and body build. However, everyone has the same anatomical structures and processes inside one's body and the same regulative functions that keep all human beings alive. The elements of balance—adaptation, homeostasis, equilibrium, needs, and health—are universally present in order to survive. Behavior is the linchpin that unleashes the forces of balance to enable us all to survive.

What makes people behave differently and why do they react the same way at times? What dictates those similar behaviors and what accounts for differences? What is behavior?

Behavior in organisms is basically defined as its actions in response to its environment.[1] Certain animal behaviors result from instinct, such as nesting, while others, such as hunting, must be learned. Movements of organic and inorganic particles within the body behave in a particular fashion following the principles of science, and these are also termed behavior. In human beings, behavior takes on a different meaning when viewed in the context of their environment, both internal and external, taking into consideration the myriad factors that influence behavior. Culture plays a dominant influence on people's behavior. Stress influences behavior in a multitude of ways. Differences in reaction to the same stimuli or stressor vary from one individual to another. Personality, gender, and maturational stage are among those factors that also influence behavior.

In this chapter, we examine those behaviors of human beings in their struggle to survive. More importantly, we identify the role of balance in human behavior and some of the ways that people maintain balance, whether instinctively or through the learning process. We hope to develop an understanding of **balance-seeking** as a common denominator of the human being's innate need for survival and beyond the basic human need into the higher realms of human behavior that are psychologically determined.

All behaviors contain the element of action, which means that something must have triggered the movement. In essence, a force or stimuli must be present in order to generate a reaction, the response. A response is the energy that changes the direction of the stimuli in one direction, or in the opposite direction. The response could be beneficial to the body, or cause harm. The response could be adaptive, which benefits the human being, or cause negative consequences such as allergic reactions. Stimuli could be anything generated internally inside the body of the organism, or from the outside or external environment. Man as a biologic organism is subject to numerous stimuli in its internal and external environments. But rather than looking at behavior as simply stimuli-response actions, we find that human behavior is much more complex. Behavioral response in different individuals; even with the same stimuli or situations, can be quite unpredictable.

On the other hand, the predictability of a person's reaction to a stimuli cannot be totally generalized. There are certain behaviors that are predictable because they are instinctive. For instance, reflexive withdrawal of a finger from the flame of a candle is a universal reaction. Breathing rapidly to compensate for decreased supply of air is instinctive and physiologically driven. A startled reaction to a loud noise is reflexive and does not require thought. People drink fluids when they are thirsty; they eat food when they are hungry; they seek shelter when they are exposed to the harsh elements of nature; they exhibit pain behaviors when subjected to painful stimuli. These behaviors are directly observable and can be described. Or, the person can also describe the sensations that triggered the stimuli. Although the goals of these behaviors are common human goals, the manner in which these behaviors are exhibited differ individually or among groups of people. Over time, culture has altered the way that people meet these needs. Modern man has "refined" eating behaviors compared to that of the pre-historic man eating meat in the jungle.

Instinct by definition is the innate tendency in animals that is inheritable and unalterable by its very nature. Basically, these instinctive behaviors have been passed on biologically throughout human existence. The biological need for air, water, nutrition, safety, and reproduction have persisted as instincts in order for the human species to survive. These are what Abraham Maslow had identified as the basic human needs and these needs have to be met first in the order for survival. Once the basic physiologic human needs are met, then the psychological needs emerge and become the more dominant determinant of behavior. Psychological needs also have physical basis in the way that the human brain works. The explanation of how the brain responds to these psychological urges is still a largely uncharted domain in modern science. Human needs are elements of balance identified earlier in the book as essential to survival.

Not all stimuli can influence the organism in order to affect behavior. Some stimuli may not be strong enough to produce a reaction and overcome its **inertia**, the tendency for an object to stay at rest until a force exerts energy on it to make it move. Distance could also be a factor in this equation. The Newtonian principles of motion[8] appear to be operational in these instances. A stimulus may have energy but if the individual does not perceive it as significant, then he/she does not react to it. The stimulus may or may not be essential to survival. For instance, a person who is emotionally disturbed or has strong reasons not to eat, placing food in front of a person may not necessarily make him or her eat. Not eating for a lengthy period will threaten survival. This creates a physiologic imbalance. The need for food (stimulus) has to be strong enough to make the individual eat. This behavior, a response to a physiologic need returns the person to a state of balance. Distance and lack of access to food would also influence food-seeking behavior. Humans during its history, have travelled long distances and caused migration shifts because of the human need to search for food supplies. In fact, this is an adaptive behavior to adjust to environmental conditions. Animals in Antarctic regions eat massive amounts of food to prepare for the anticipated scarcity of food during the winter months.

THEORETICAL FOUNDATIONS: RELEVANT THEORIES OF HUMAN BEHAVIOR

To understand human behavior, it is important to look at modern theories that have served as foundations to the practice of the health care and mental health professions. The list of human behavioral theorists is long but only those that are relevant to the concept of balance will be mentioned in this chapter. Their works have been classified into categories such as Systems Theory, Behaviorism & Social Learning Theory, Family Systems, Psychodynamic Theory, Psychosocial Development Theory, Transpersonal Theory, Social Exchange Theory, Social Constructionism, Symbolic Interactionism, Conflict Theory, and Contingency Theory.[3,4] A brief overview of the following theorists will be discussed: Pavlov's Classic Conditioning Theory,[2] Freud's Psychoanalytic Theory,[2] Talcott Parson's Actions Systems,[5] Erikson's Psychosocial Development Theory,[2] Maslow's Humanistic Psychology Theory and Hierarchy of Needs,[2] and Bowen's Family Systems.[6]

Ivan Pavlov (1849-1936) was Russian physiologist who developed his famous Classical Conditioning Theory from his experiments with dogs. He noticed that the dogs began to salivate when they anticipated that food would be forthcoming. Then he found that when the food that triggered the stimulation was paired with a neutral stimulus (a bell), that the sound of the bell alone could elicit salivation in the dogs. These observations led him to develop the stimulus-response concept or respondent conditioning of behavior. This concept focused on the belief that behavior can be influenced by a process called conditioning. This forms the basis for his Classical Conditioning Theory. The limitation of his work was that it represented physiological responses without the psychological component of behavior. However, his experiments opened the way for other behavioral theories. As a behavioral model, it emphasized that observable behavioral responses are learned and can be modified in an environment.

Sigmund Freud (1856-1939) was born in 1856 to a businessman father. He was the oldest of eight children and had a very close relationship with his mother, who was considered his mother's favorite. Sigmund Freud developed his groundbreaking theory of personality structure, levels of awareness, anxiety, the role of defense mechanisms and anxiety in people's lives. His theory revolutionized the thinking about mental health disorders and developed techniques that are still used to this day. His identification of conscious and unconscious influences on human behavior provided basis for using individual "talk therapy", known as the cathartic method, frequently used as a technique in identifying clients' problems. He is known for his three levels of awareness: the id, the ego, and the superego.[2,7]

The **id** is the unconscious and the most primitive part of the personality. It is present at birth and the source of all drives, instincts, reflexes, needs, genetic inheritance. It is based on the pleasure principle that seeks instant gratification in order to satisfy needs, minimize pain, and maximize pleasure. The id cannot tolerate frustration and seeks release of tension. Tension is discharged through behaviors that are reflexive and automatic, such as gagging, crying, and laughing. These behaviors alleviate some forms of tension without regard for the consequences. For instance, crying is the only way of communication and signals that the infant is hungry. The tension is the hunger drive when the infant feels the biologic need for food. If the infant does not get fed, it will continue to cry. If its hunger need is not met by giving it milk, the tension is not relieved and the infant will continue to cry. As soon as enough milk is provided, the tension is relieved and the infant will stop crying. A look of satisfaction may be visible on the infant's face after having been fed. The pleasure principle has been applied.

However, not all tension can be relieved through reflex action and this is called a state of anxiety. An infant separated from its mother feels this tension and begins to cry. The reflex action of crying does not signify a physiologic need. It indicates a psychological need of the infant to be held by its mother and the separation creates an anxiety. This tension is not relieved by food. It is the kind of tension that has produced anxiety and cannot be relieved until the source of anxiety is removed. The infant will then feel pleasure when held by the mother and anxiety is relieved. The id-dominated personality does not consider the consequences of their actions but simply the gratification of basic needs and urges.

The **ego** surfaces around the fourth or fifth month of life because the needs and demands of the id can no longer be satisfactorily met through reflex actions. The ego follows the reality principle which is now able to differentiate between subjective and the objective reality of the outside world. The ego has to master the impulses of the id to preserve itself from anxiety. The **superego**, highest level of awareness, is the last part of personality to develop. It acts as the conscience and actually delays the immediate impulses generated by the id to bring it in touch with reality and rationality. The superego represents the "ideal" rather than reality, which at times may not be congruent with each other. It is the ego that acts to balance the demands of the id and the superego. When the demands of the id and the superego conflict with each other, the ego suffers a state of anxiety and becomes a source of disorder.

Freud believed that there are five stages of human development from infancy to adulthood but much of the individual's personality develops during the first five years of life. The basic personality structure is already formed during this period and this determines the person's adjustment patterns and personality during the later stages. These psychosexual stages are: oral (0-1 yr), anal (1-3yr), phallic oedipal (3-6 yr), latency (6-12 yr), and genital (12 yr and beyond). These stages involve initially the development of trust in the environment and where needs can be met, to control of these impulses, then parental relationships, further development of skills to cope with the environment, and finally, the ability to be creative and find pleasure in relationship with others and in society where he lives.

Erik Erikson (1902-1994)[7] was an American psychoanalyst who initially was a follower of Freud but later on changed his beliefs about Freudian psychology. He believed that the Freudian theory was inherently restrictive and that culture and society play a significant role in the development of personality. Unlike Freud, Erikson believed that the development of personality covers the whole life span cycle and not limited to the first five years. His emphasis was more on social growth. He developed the eight stages of personality that are the major life cycles of individuals with developmental tasks in each stage. Successful resolution of one stage will have a positive effect on the person's personality as they grow older. Biological maturation and social influences as the person grows to adulthood are imminent changes even if the person is not able to resolve changes at each stage successfully. The eight stages of Erikson and the corresponding ages these developed are: 1. Trust vs. mistrust (0-18 mo.), 2. Autonomy vs. shame and doubt (18 mo.-3 yrs), 3. Initiative vs. guilt (3-6 yrs), 4. Industry vs. inferiority (6-11 yrs), 5. Identity vs. role confusion (11-20 yrs), 6. Intimacy vs. isolation (18-25 yrs), 7. Generativity vs. stagnation (21-45 yrs), and 8. Ego integrity vs. despair (45 yrs to death). Erikson was among the first popular psychologists to recognize the continuity of human development from childhood to adulthood and throughout the lifespan.

Abraham Maslow (1908-1970) introduced the humanistic approach to psychology and has influenced the development of other theories, especially in nursing. He introduced the concept of the hierarchy of needs discussed in the first chapter. This hierarchy of needs explained the motivation of human behavior, beginning with the most basic physiologic needs to the highest, which he called the stage of self-actualization. The first level, physiologic needs have to met first before other higher levels could be met. For instance, a person in need of air has to breathe oxygen first or suffer death. Or a starving person needs to have fluids and nutrition to survive. Inability to meet the basic physiologic needs will lead to death of the human being. The five levels of Maslow's hierarchy are first, physiologic need for air, food, water, sleep, and sex. The last has something to do with the human's ability to self-propagate his species to continue his survival on earth. This does not have immediate consequences but the other needs do. Besides sex, deprivation of those other elements will pose almost immediate danger to survival. The second level in the hierarchy is safety and security, third is love and belonging, fourth is esteem and self-esteem, and fifth is self-actualization.

It is the **self-actualization** level where Maslow concentrated much of his work, studying "self-actualized" famous people, some dead and some living at the time of his study like Abraham Lincoln, Thomas Jefferson, Walt Whitman, Beethoven, William James, Eleanor Roosevelt, Albert Einstein, and Albert Schweitzer. According to Maslow, some characteristics of self-actualized persons include such behavioral manifestations as [2]: an accurate perception of reality; acceptance of themselves, others and nature; problem-centered rather than self-centered orientation; active social interest; democratic character structure (display little racial, religious, or social prejudice); autonomy, independence and self-sufficient; and creativity, especially in managing their lives.

Talcott Parson's Action Systems (1902-1979), was an American psychologist who was raised with a strong Protestant background and later taught at Harvard University from 1927-1973.[9] He is well known for his work with structural functionalism, his action system theory and the AGIL scheme (acronym for adaptation, goal attainment, integration, and latency). Parsons developed a "grand theory" for the analysis of society based on a structural-functional approach. His approach is based on his four action systems: Social system, Cultural system, Personality system, and Behavioral organism.

In Parson's view, society is a structure with interrelated parts but functions as a whole with its constituent elements of norms, customs, traditions, and institutions. Function is a complex of activities that are directed towards meeting a need or the needs of a system. His is a major theory of a body of work on the theory of human behavior that focuses on systems.

Systems theories focus on how persons interact with their environment. In Parson's AGIL scheme, adaptation means that a system must adapt to its environment; goal attainment is that the system must define and achieve its primary goals; integration is that the system has interrelationship with its other parts to maintain the whole; and latency is that the system maintains and renews the motivation of individuals and the cultural patterns that create and sustain these motivations[5].

His theory focuses on the relationship between man and his environment and society—it influences him and he influences and changes it. Culture plays a major role in binding the major elements of society. It mediates interactions among "actors" or human beings, their personality development, and the social systems that arise from these interactions. Adaptation is a requirement for a system to thrive. For a social system to survive, functional prerequisites must be met—it must have support of the other systems, meet the needs of the actors, and control over disruptions in the system. Personality is not only controlled by the cultural system but also by social system. Behavior is the source of energy for the rest of the system. Without behavior, the system would not be able to adapt and thrive.

Bowen's Systems Theory of the Family. Murray Bowen, MD (1931-1990) was born in a small town of Waverly, Tennessee. After obtaining his medical degree, he became a professor of Psychiatry at Georgetown University and later became the first director of the Family Division of the National Institute of Mental Health (NIMH). The Bowen family systems theory is a theory of human behavior that places **the** family as the center of emotional systems that govern human relationships since the beginning of its existence. He developed eight concepts in his Family Systems Theory[6,10] Bowen believed that emotional systems beginning with the family has evolved over the millions of years of human existence. In his view, family members differ in their level of emotional maturity and produced variations among family members. These differences are transmitted across generations as the individual learns to adapt within the family unit over the generations. Sibling position also plays a role in their development. It is the connectedness of the members of the family that promotes emotional interdependence. This interdependence evolved to promote the cooperation and teamwork required to protect, shelter, and nourish their members. Increased levels of tension can also occur in the family that can lead to anxiety and can spread among them. As the tension increases, it can overwhelm one or all family members. Emotional systems also govern behavior on the societal level.

The cornerstone of the Bowen Family Systems Theory is contained in his eight basic concepts briefly described here:

1. Levels of differentiation of self—Individuals vary in their thinking based on their concept of the "self". The person's functioning is influenced to a larger or lesser degree

in the individual's ability to exert control over themselves or on others, and conform to the group.

2. The nuclear family—This concept describes relationship patterns that develop in the family and the problems that may develop.

3. Family projection process—This concept describes the way parents transmit their emotional problems on their child/children and may negatively affect them.

4. Multigenerational transmission process—This focuses on the way that differences in family relationships are transmitted across generations.

5. Sibling position—This is based on the belief that people who have the same sibling position may develop some important common characteristics.

6. Triangles—This considers the triangle, a three-person relationship system, as the most stable relationship. It can manage tension better as tension is distributed among the three, such as the third as the neutral party in a conflict.

7. Emotional cut off—When people have emotional conflicts with others in the family and they cut off emotional contact with them, which does not resolve the conflict.

8. Societal emotional process—Describes how emotional systems governs behavior on a societal level.

Various theories of behavior, including the ones just described, underscore the multiple facets of behavior. It could be on the physiological, psychological, socio-cultural level, or all of these. The complexity of human behavior cannot be overstated. It is the prime instrument of survival. The theories of Maslow, Pavlov, Freud, Erikson, Parsons, and Bowen have given greater understanding of the myriads of ways and factors that influence behavior. In Pavlov's stimuli-response theory, the physiologic response is emphasized, manifested by the dog salivating as a conditioned response to the bell. Physiologic responses are also elicited by stress in stress responses, such as the Selye's "fight or flight" reaction, the stimulation of the sympathetic nerves that generate physiologic changes, and the gradual return to equilibrium when the stress is resolved or when the individual adjusts to it. This is the process of adaptation that is also an element in the theories of Parsons and Bowen.

Adaptation is an important element of behavior that has been recognized by theorists although in different ways. Parsons' theory of structural functionalism views society as a whole in terms of its cultural elements, such as norms, traditions, customs, and institutions. It looks at behavior from the standpoint of the society where persons live and the systems that are operating to sustain them in the environment. Function is directed towards meeting a need, or the need of a system. Adaptation, the first in the AGIL system is required in order for human beings to adjust to its environment. Bowen looks at adaptation within the family unit as the actors deal with emotional, biological and environmental influences. It is the ability to adapt within the family unit and find the balance between the influences of others and their own selves that enable them to transmit patterns across generations.

Theoretical relevance to balance

Personality plays a key role in human behaviors. The influence of the mind on personality has also been a subject of intense study. Among the first to develop this concept of the influence of the mind on human behavior was Freud. The three levels of awareness, the id, ego and superego, appear to parallel Maslow's hierarchy of needs. The id which is present in all human beings at birth, responds only to basic human needs of air, food, water, elimination. Behavior at this level is reflexive and requires instant gratification for survival. The ego develops about six months after birth and continues along with the development of the superego, the last level to develop. The ego serves both the id and superego. In Maslow's model, the psychological needs emerge once the basic and lower needs are met. Safety and security needs have to be met first before belongingness, self esteem, and finally, self-actualization. According to Freud, the individual's personality is already fully developed at an early age, as opposed to that of Erikson who viewed personality development as happening over a lifetime. Maslow's self-actualization stage could be compared to a fully developed superego of Freud. However, self-actualization is a characteristic of mature adults, not found among children.

Balance is the dynamic interplay of the essential elements within a system to achieve a state of stability. This interplay requires energy and movement, whether it happens internally or outwardly. This is called behavior. Behavior is required to achieve balance through its basic elements of adaptation, homeostasis, equilibrium, fulfillment of needs, and health. The human being functions within an open system that has an intake capacity for stimuli and an output mechanism to produce a response. All processes within this system requires behavior or movement observable or measurable, within the internal and external environment. The purpose of behavior is ultimately to achieve balance and equilibrium within the person ensuring his survival. The body is already quipped internally to achieve physiologic balance, a common denominator among all human beings. External manifestations of behavior is a response to stimuli from within or from the outside. For example, a person who is thirsty is driven by this innate need to seek and drink water. Drinking water is an observable external behavior, in response to a basic need but stimulated by the thirst mechanism inside the body. This thirst mechanism is controlled by the central command, the brain. The goal of this behavior is to seek balance, created by an imbalance that triggered the thirst response. Once the person's thirst is quenched, the body acts to dampen the response, a negative feedback mechanism, so that the person stops drinking. Homeostatic equilibrium has been restored and the body is again in a state of balance.

In Maslow's theory, psychological needs emerge once the basic physiologic needs have been met. In Freud's theory, the ego and superego dominates over the id, once the id's needs have been satisfied. Psychological needs are much more complicated and difficult to measure.

Beyond the simple stimulus-response perspective of Pavlov, psychological needs take into consideration the role of the psyche, the mental faculties that make us all unique human beings. But psychological development follows maturational sequence according to Erikson. According to Bowen, the family plays a major role in the development of personality and so does culture. In Parson's view, human development happens within a system or interrelated systems and structures that work together to support people's survival. Behavior within the system includes adaptation of the person to its environment. Social systems, need to be supported by culture, personality, and adaptive behaviors. It is the behavioral system that handles the adaptation function by adjusting to its changes. By so doing, the environment is also changed.

The emergence of psychological needs follow the basic survival needs. Maslow has differentiated the various levels of psychological needs in a hierarchy. It appears that these needs are innate to human beings but the manner in which they are manifested in terms of behavior varies from one individual to another, even within the same family due to factors that Bowen postulated in his theory. The nuclear family from which human beings originated serves as the source of safety and security, love and sense of belonging, and supported his self-esteem. Communication became a means for human beings to have common understanding in interactions with others. The development of language is outside the scope of this book. Patterns of interactions within the family and communications used to relate with others became part of the culture that get passed on from generation to generation.

The balance of the influences of the internal factors and external influences on behavior then becomes clearer. When individuals find balance of these factors, they become more self-actualizing (Maslow). They achieve a state of equilibrium that is conducive to well-being and continued survival. A state of optimal physical and mental well-being, and not merely the absence of disease is called health, as defined by the World Health Organization. The behavior that enables human beings to adapt to their environment, seek fulfillment of their physiological and psychological needs, and attain a level of well-being, pleasure, and self-fulfillment is called **balance-seeking.** Ultimately, the goal of balance-seeking behavior is survival by meeting the requirements of the elements of balance: adaptation, equilibrium, homeostasis, needs, and health. This behavior is as individual as every human being on this planet. The external factors that affect this behavior include family dynamics, society, and culture. Importantly, it is how individuals process these factors in their brain and decide how to respond to it. In Freud's view, the ego acts to balance the influences of the id and the superego. Inability to find this balance can cause anxiety and emotional problems. Coping mechanisms will enable the person to restore emotional balance and well-being.

Behavior can also automatic and reflexive and does not require thought, like the instantaneous withdrawal of a finger by the person when exposed to intense heat. It could also be observed in the instinctive avoidance of an object you see falling in your direction. This behavior does not require mental processing. It serves one immediate purpose: to protect and ensure survival at the basic level. Automatic physiological responses are also forms of behavior that happen internally. The movement of fluids, electrolytes, oxygen, carbon dioxide, nutrients, and elements of the blood all participate in the behavioral process of maintaining the body's internal homeostatic functions. This movement, although not directly observable, could be measured at any particular time by modern laboratory instruments. This gives a snapshot picture of the state of physiologic equilibrium of the body at a given time.

MIND AND MATTER

How does the mind control behavior? The human mind, the source of ideas, thoughts, feelings and emotions has been studied for a long time. The search for a better understanding of the mind and the role it plays in behavior and all its manifestations, such as emotions and feelings have been a source of fascination for thinking humans throughout the ages. Despite all the theories of human behaviors, particularly advanced by the science of psychology, sociology and psychiatry, a lot more are left to be desired. It is like the proverbial fruit that is too out of reach to be eaten. Huge leaps have been made in discovering the functions of the different parts of the brain and mental processes. However, many questions are still left unanswered. Going back to the evolutionary time when this giant leap was made between a non-thinking animal being to a thinking intelligent human being continues to be mainly a scientific conjecture.

What we now know in the science of anatomy and physiology will help us understand the mind and its functions to infer how it give rise to psychological and mental behavioral manifestations.

It is important to point out the role of the nervous system in the development of mind and behavior. Mind cannot be separated from matter. The human brain is often likened to a computer. However, no matter how sophisticated the most advanced computer is, no man has been able to duplicate the intricate functions of the brain. It is the part of the body that enables it to function intellectually, control physiological responses, maintain basic life support systems, process psychological stimuli, and consciously or unconsciously dictate how we behave. The brain is divided into three major components: the cerebrum, brain stem and the cerebellum. The **cerebrum** is further composed of two identical-looking hemispheres: the left hemisphere and the right hemisphere. Both hemispheres are further divided into four main lobes: frontal, temporal, parietal, and occipital. The **frontal lobe** is said to control higher cognitive functions, memory and retention, voluntary eye and motor movement, and expressive speech. It is believed that this segment of the brain is responsible for **personality** development. Personality is what defines each human being as unique. Personality factors include, not only physical attributes, but also inherited traits, genetic make-up, cultural influences and adaptive capacities.

The **neuron** is the basic structure that compose the nervous system. Neurons detect changes in the environment and initiate body responses to maintain a dynamic steady state.[12] In order for the neurons to function, it needs energy derived from food sources, primarily glucose and fatty acids. Oxygen is vital during the complex process of cell respirations in which energy is released. The neurons have the function of receiving and transmitting impulses from one part of the body to another. To preserve brain function, the integrity of the neurons need to be ensured. The exquisite and intricate functions of each cell in the body, including the nerve cells, all work interrelatedly to form a harmonious functioning of all the body parts in the human being. Without this wholeness and integrity, there can be no learning and no life on this planet can exist.

In the evolutionary process, the control of basic vital functions is housed in the earliest part of the brain to develop: **the brain stem**. The brain stem links the newer parts of the brain, the cerebral hemispheres with the thalamus and the limbic system. It is in the cerebral hemispheres, left and right, that created man's intellect and will. The limbic system organizes moods, memory, and appetites. The brain stem connects with the most primitive part of the nervous system within the spinal cord. It also serves as the major highway for motor and sensory impulses to conduct information to and from the brain. These structures are bathed in a clear fluid called the cerebrospinal fluid that circulates throughout the nervous system.

For the brain stem to develop first is logical because without it, human beings could not survive. It houses vital centers that control breathing, heart rate, blood pressure, and level of consciousness. Deep within the brain stem is the cluster of cells called the reticular formation within which lies the basic life support systems. Knocking out this function will wipe out life of the human being. This life support system needs a constant barrage of information from within the body. Because of its central location, the reticular formation receives information from all parts of the body so that it could make adjustments to changes that occur. These adjustments are made continually by the body, whether asleep or awake.

A cluster of nerve cells in the **reticular formation** controls the stomach, mouth, face, ears and eyes. Sensations from these organs are fed through this group of cells that control their output from the brain stem and forms part of consciousness. The cells controlling consciousness form a chain that runs through the center of the brain stem to the midbrain, then these impulses spread to the right and left cerebral hemispheres. Nervous fibers in the **cerebral cortex** when stimulated are also able to excite other groups of large cells so that the cerebral cortex can start processing information. Combined with information from memory, emotional and feeling states from the limbic system, all these information are synthesized to form the world of consciousness.[11]

The **cerebrum** is the seat of consciousness, metal processes, learning, speech, thought, and recall of all humans. The frontal lobe of the cerebrum is thought to have the greatest influence on the development of personality, the quality which makes each person a unique being. There are so many theories of personality but it is doubtful that there is one single theory that could account for the complex nature of man. There are two halves of the brain: the right hemisphere and the left hemisphere. Although they are physically identical, their functions are totally different. The left hemisphere is specifically involved in inference, deduction and language, while the right hemisphere is responsible for spatial orientation, artistic ability, creativity, musical ability, and appreciation of color and shapes. Despite the duality of these two hemispheres, they connect with each other so that the brain functions as a whole.

The physical origins of learning and memory that compose a major part of who we are as intelligent beings are still being studied and explored. Learning from experiences enable human beings to store information as memory. Ivan Pavlov, the Russian scientist, described learning in terms of basic units of behavior called conditional reflexes. But more complicated learning happens in the higher center in the cerebrum. The learning process is important in the study of human behavior. Language is one of the skills learned by humans that lower animals don't. This acquired skill is probably one of the greatest leap in the evolutionary process. Through language, we learn from our experiences and pass this on to others and the next generations. Language is an embodiment of culture and enables humans to establish linguistic connections with and influence other humans.

Emotions are part of human behavior that are consciously experienced and cause psychological stress as well as physiological reactions. Emotions are felt in a whole variety of ways and intensity. Usually, emotions are in response to immediate situations but even events from some time ago could also evoke emotional responses. Hedonic feelings, or feelings of pleasantness and unpleasantness are the most fundamental emotional experiences.[11] Joy, laughter, love, and contentment evoke pleasant feelings and are considered positive. On the other hand, fear, grief, hate and resentment are unpleasant or negative experiences. Some emotional responses are modified by culture, personality and past experiences. The physical basis for emotions is even harder to pinpoint. The limbic system, situated in the inner portion of the midbrain near the base of the brain, apparently plays a crucial role in emotional status and psychological function.[13] Stimulation of the limbic system can evoke emotions, feelings and behaviors that ensure survival and self-preservation. Extreme emotional feelings such as fear and grief, are accompanied by physiological changes in the body. In a highly emotional state, the body prepares itself for **"fight or flight"**, the first signal of which comes from the brain. Adrenaline is released which triggers a series of interrelated physiological responses in the body. These physiological responses disturb the normal body equilibrium and throws it into imbalance. After a period of time, the tendency of the body is to go back to its natural state of equilibrium through processes that decrease the adrenaline response.

ADAPTATION AND BEHAVIOR

The human race would not have survived as a species without having adapted to the internal and external influences that always impinge upon its physical and psychological self. Adaptation is defined as the adjustment of an organism to a change in internal or external conditions or circumstances.[14] The concept of adaptation was used by a nursing theorist Sister Callista Roy in her Adaptation Model. The goal of nursing according to Roy, is to promote adaptive physiological, self-concept, role function, and interdependent responses. During the early prehistoric life of man, climatic changes have made adaptation imperative for it to survive the harsh environment where they lived. The need for food in the hash arid African desert or the frozen Siberian tundra where the early humans found themselves, have made adaptation critical to their survival. Even much earlier in the evolutionary process, humans developed larger brains, walked more upright, developed fine motor skills and vocal signal graduated into speech.[15] According to studies, the brain of the prehistoric modern human developed rapidly outside the womb. Intense selective pressures must have been exerted on the genes controlling the development of their brains and these pressures are in the form of intellectual development. As the brain was developing, the motor skills to use tools and vocal signals that evolved into speech patterns were also evolving. As a result, interactions among other humans were progressively becoming more complicated. This made the environment richer and more varied. The changing social and physical environment as the world was approaching the Ice Age must have furthered this evolutionary process. In the words of one scientist, Christopher Wills on this evolutionary development of the brain, ". . . as the pace of social and cultural evolution accelerated, the environment of each generation became progressively more and more different from the environment of those preceding it . . . ."[18]

Adaptation is the key to evolution. This capacity to adapt by managing and manipulating the environment to serve their needs enabled man to survive. Developing ancient tools for hunting and fishing were adaptive behaviors. More than ordinary animals without well-developed brains, the human beings, became more superior and emerged better at survival. The better adapted they are, the more successful they become as the move up the evolutionary chain. This adaptive behavior remains one of our greatest assets as human beings. The effects of evolution continue as long as man survives. Adaptive behaviors need a balancing of the internal and external environment to promote his survival and well-being. As a highly developed being in the continuous march through evolution, man will have to adapt to life on this planet.

Adaptive behaviors

Adaptive behaviors are responses that have been encoded in the person's pattern of responses to consistent and persistent stimuli. The ultimate goal of adaptive behavior is survival. Human beings since the beginning of time have changed their patterns of behavior to meet their basic needs for survival. This is because of the human mind, housed in a well-developed brain that make us different from other animals with only complex physical adaptations. "In a sense, we are biologically adapted to adapt"[16] according to Spencer Wells, a genetic scientist famous for his work that contributed to understanding of human prehistory. Our adaptations come in the form of behavioral changes. According to Wells, the development of culture is one of the results of having a highly adaptive mind. The mind, as we have seen, is responsible for our psychological responses. Humans are able to think because of its superior physical characteristic: the human brain. The brain dictates our physiologic responses to keep the internal equilibrium, essential for survival. It does so without bidding because of the body's innate ability to maintain internal equilibrium, an element of balance. This interrelationship between the body and the mind is what makes us complex beings a more simple whole.

Adaptation will continue as long as human beings exist on this planet. Without adaptation, the human species could not survive. It is adaptive behaviors in response to internal and external changes in our environments that enable us to evolve continually. The key to evolution is the concept of adaptation.[17] We know from modern scientific discoveries that the evolution of man to a bi-pedal intelligent being enabled it to find better sources of food, develop and manipulate tools, and on the whole, manage environmental changes. Furthermore, intelligence enabled human beings to establish and pass on culture as a social being.

It is often said that man is a social animal. Well, modern humans really are. We don't really know conclusively even to this day, what led to this extraordinary development of man as a social being. The maternal instinct to nurture their young perhaps contributed to the basic social relationship. Contributing to it is the relatively long period of maturational development of the young that enabled it to acquire more information and skills over a longer period of time. It probably really began with the basic instinctive sexual behavior, nature's way of self-propagation of the species. Social groups probably became a necessity as a means of protecting their own kind and surviving the harsh environment where early humans found themselves. Unlike other animals with less intellectual capacity, humans used this advantage to become more organized and thrive. Wherever humans spread themselves all over the world, they carried with them the capacity for adaptation and with it, the development of other social skills for survival and better lives. Such physical and mental behavioral adaptations have apparently led to the development of different societies and cultures. With the help of their developing linguistic capability and diversity, many different cultures evolved as we see them today.

THE BEHAVIOR PYRAMID MODEL

Using Maslow's Hierarchy of Needs and the developmental patterns found in Sigmund Freud's and Erickson's theories as basis for the model, I developed a **Behavior Pyramid Model** of Realms of Behavior which I classified into four levels: (see Behavior Pyramid Diagram)

1. Reflexive or automatic realm
2. Emotional /Spiritual realm
3. Intellectual/Rational realm
4. Self-fulfillment and Balance realm

The **reflexive or automatic realm** is that level of behavior where the focus is the satisfaction of basic human needs and the preservation of safety and security. Behavior does not require thought. It is purely a direct response to a stimuli with the function of enabling survival and protection of the physical integrity of the body. This level has a physical basis in the development of the human brain. Freud's id level of awareness and Maslow's first level of his hierarchy are operational here because this is where the human being's basic human needs are met: air, water, food, elimination, and sex. This behavior is at the primordial level that we share in common with lower species in the animal kingdom. Reflexive responses are in the unconscious or semi-conscious level and respond to basic survival needs and protection. These are present at birth but also continue throughout life. These needs have the highest priority for survival. Safety and security are needs that also belong to this level because lack of it or deprivation of, will also directly threaten survival. In Erickson's developmental theory, this is the stage of trust vs. mistrust. Infants have their needs met through those individuals who they trust will provide them with their needs for the moment. The infant is completely dependent on others to meet their basic needs.

The **emotional/spiritual realm** is where psychological needs start to emerge. Emotions are generated as a later feature of the human brain, the limbic system in the mid-brain. At this level, the individual's brain has matured enough to develop the ego, to temper the primal impulses of the id. Babies are now able to control some of their reflexive impulses and there is more cognition on their part to appreciate reality. Social pressures begin to be appreciated by the child as the emotional level develops. Developing physical and mental abilities enable children to explore the world around them. The developing young person seeks love and belonging from those significant people in their lives, especially the family. This is where Bowen's Theory of Family Systems become more important. Relationships within the nuclear family plays an important role in nurturing the maturing individual. The level of differentiation between the family and others in social groups begin to be felt more. Love and a sense of belonging are needs that become more paramount as the individual continues in the socialization process. External and internal influences become more profound. The external influences include the social and physical environment such as culture and society, the environment, and nature; internal influences include inherited traits, personality, maturational factors, and mental well-being. A growing sense of autonomy can come in direct conflict with family needs and values and the individual tries to seek balance between these pulls of influences.

Spiritual needs become integrated as part of the person's development, or this might come later in a person's life. Values of right and wrong, the mores of the culture, and the belief in a higher power become part of the belief system. These beliefs are part of the cultural patterns of behavior that are inculcated in the young person's mind and become their moral compass. Religious behaviors observed and practiced by the family are integrated into the member's behavior, such as going to religious services, praying at certain times of the day or occasions. Rituals of the dying or dead, as part of religious practices are seen and observed and engrained in the young person's mind. In some cultures, such as the Native American Indian tribes, where harmony with nature is a strong part of their belief, this is part of their spiritual development. Spirituality or religious beliefs play a stabilizing effect on the person. During times of stress, such as death, separation, divorce, or illness, turning to a higher power for solace and hope provides inner peace and balance and enables mobilization of coping mechanisms. Spirituality as a psychosocial need, is also important in seeking inner balance in an increasingly stressful and complex society. Research have shown the important link among the mind, body and spirit. A person's health depends on a balance of physical, psychological, sociological, cultural, developmental and spiritual factors.[17]

Spirituality and religion are often used synonymously but these two terms are not the same. Spirituality is an awareness of one's inner self and a sense of connection with a power greater than themselves. Research has shown the important link between the mind, body and spirit. It is the way we connect with a Being greater than ourselves and the world, and the universe. It gives meaning and purpose to the lives of those persons with a high sense of spirituality. On the other hand, religion is a belief in a specific deity or god that rules the world and from where we obtain guidance, strength, and purpose. There are so many different religions in various cultures of the world and it is in fact, an element of culture. Spirituality is an important factor that often helps in achieving balance to maintain health and well-being.

The **intellectual/rational realm** is when the individual reaches physical and emotional maturity so that he/she is able to meet basic needs on their own, find safety and security, and love and belonging in their interrelationships within the social structure. Culture and its component elements, such as language, values, beliefs, and spirituality have found a niche in the superego, where it is actively being balanced by the ego. In the physical development of the brain, the person may have either a dominant left brain or right brain, or a combination of both. Logical thought and reasoning and the achievement of creativity can now be more fully achieved at this level, along with maturational development. Self-esteem is now occupying a higher importance, perhaps superseding other emotional needs at times. A healthy self-esteem is necessary for the individual to achieve developmental goals at this stage. Having nurtured family members, the individual passes on to the stage where cultural values and collective knowledge acquired from previous generations are also passed on to the next. The wisdom of the older generation reaches greater importance if the following generations are to continue their psychological and mental development. This is possible when the social systems support this transmission of culture. According to Parson's Action System theory, culture is the major force binding the various elements of the social world through evolutionary changes and adaptive behaviors.

The **Self-fulfillment and Balance realm** is the highest level of human behavior achievable. It is equivalent to Maslow's Self-Actualization level where the individual has reached his highest potential. However, my view of self-fulfillment is that this is the level where the individual feels the highest form of balance in their lives. Although it may be a factor, achievement and success in their occupation or profession is only one aspect. It is the totality of the person's experience that matters. All their needs are met to a certain degree that brings a sense of well-being and wholeness. All the elements of balance are lined up and operating to maintain his entire system. Spiritual needs are fulfilled at this level, which do not refer to any one particular organized religion. It is his personal relationship with a higher power where spiritual fulfillment is achieved. A self-fulfilled person may not necessarily enjoy the best of physical health. A self-fulfilled person is in a state of optimal physical, emotional, mental, and spiritual well-being in balance with each other to maintain wholeness.

Balance-seeking behaviors

In the Behavior Pyramid Model, balance must be achieved at every level for the person to continue surviving and thriving as a social being in the modern world. This is achieved through balance-seeking behaviors. In this model, balance-seeking behaviors are those unconscious and/or conscious actions to meet physiologic, physical, and psychosocial needs to maintain equilibrium. Balance-seeking behaviors are performed at every level of the Behavior Pyramid in the person's life. Balance-seeking during childhood, is meeting the basic human needs for survival and safety. As psycho-social needs acquire greater role and importance in a person's life, balance-seeking takes the form of those behaviors to secure love, belongingness, acceptance within the social structure of the culture where the person lives. As the person expands his interrelationship with others in society and acquires varied roles, his self-esteem grows. Validation of his worth as a contributing member of society happens within the social structure. However, as the individual becomes more and more immersed in the society where he lives, stresses mount that could destabilize his physical and emotional balance. Stresses have a disruptive effect on the body, physiologically and emotionally, leading to imbalance. Balance-seeking behaviors will help restore the person to his normal state of balance.

*Balance—seeking behaviors will be discussed further in the next chapter

KEY CONCEPTS
• •

1. Behavior is a universal characteristic of all living humans and animals on this planet. In human beings, it is the linchpin that enables forces of the elements of balance to be manifested.
2. All behaviors contain the element of action and energy. It could be manifested internally and externally, whether under conscious control or reflexive action by the nervous system. The central nervous system is primarily responsible for the functions of those structures that generate thought, learning, emotions, that in turn determine a major aspect of personality.
3. Behavior is affected by physiological, psychological, and physical factors in the internal and external environment. It has its origins in the physical body in response to internal and external stimuli and behaviorally manifested.
4. Theories of human behavior and personality by Pavlov, Freud, Erikson, Maslow, Parsons, and Bowen provide the theoretical framework for the concept of behavior as a force of balance.
5. Balance-seeking behaviors enable human beings to adapt to their environment, seek fulfillment of their physiologic and psychological needs, attain an optimum level of well-being, and achieve full self-fulfillment. Ultimately, balance-seeking behaviors will contribute to, and promote growth and survival.
6. Adaptation is the adjustment of an organism to change in the internal and external conditions. The ultimate goal of adaptive behavior is survival.
7. The Behavior Pyramid Model has been developed based on theories by Maslow, Freud and Erikson in a hierarchy of needs from the most basic to the highest level. These levels are: 1. Reflexive or automatic, 2). Emotional, 3) Intellectual/rational, 4) Self-Fulfillment level.
8. Balance-seeking behaviors must be performed at every level of the Behavior Pyramid to continue surviving and thriving as a social being in modern society.

CHAPTER 3: BALANCE AND BEHAVIOR

REFERENCES

1. The American Heritage Science Dictionary. 2005. copyright by Houghton Miffin Company.Published by Houghton Miffin Company

2. Carson, V.B. and Trubowitz, J. 2006. "Relevant Theories and Therapies for Nursing Practice". in *Foundations of Psychiatric Mental Health Nursing* by Varcarolis, E.M.,et al. (5th ed.) St. Louis, Missouri. Saunders Elsevier.

3. Hutchison, E.D. 2003. *Dimensions of Human Behavior: Person and Environment* (2nd ed.) Thousand Oaks. Sage.

4. Robbins, S., Chatterjee, P. and Canda,E. (Eds.)2005. *Contemporary Human Behavior Theory: A Critical Perspective for Social Work* (2nd ed.) Boston. Allyn and Bacon.

5. Actions System/Crimson Locker Online: http://crimsonlockeronline.com/talcott-parsons-actions-system. retrieved 4/30/2012

6. Bowen Center-Bowen Theory. http://psychology.about.com/od/psychosocialtheories/a/psychosocial.html. retrieved 4/30/2012

7. George, J.B. 2002. "Theory as a Basis for Practice". in *Psychiatric Mental Health Nursing* (2nd ed.)Albany, New York. Delmar

8. Kauffman III, W.J. and Freedman, R.A. 1999. "Gravitation and the Motions of the Planet". in *Universe* (5th ed.) New York. W.H. Freeman and Company.

9. Talcott Parsons—New World Encyclopedia. http://www.newworldencyclopedia.org/entry/Talcott_Parsons.html. retrieved 6/18/2012.

10. Murray Bowen, M.D. and the Nine Concepts in Family Systems Theory. http://ideastoaction.wordpress.com/dr-bowen/. retrieved 6/19/2012

11. Rayner, C. (cont. Ed.) 1980. *Atlas of the Body and Mind*. Chicago, Illinois. Rand McNally & Company.

12. Huether, S. & McCance, K. (2008). "Structure and Function of the Neurologic System". in *Understanding Pathophysiology* (4th ed.) St. Louis, Missouri. Mosby Elsevier.

13. Raynor, J. 2006. "Biological Basis for Understanding Psychotropic Drugs". in *Foundations of Psychiatric Mental Health Nursing*. Varcarolis, E.M.,et al. (5th ed.) St. Louis, Missouri. Saunders Elsevier.

14. Venes, D. (Ed). 2005. *Taber's Cyclopedic Medical Dictionary* (20th ed.) Philadelphia. FA Davis Company.

15. Wills, C. 1993. *The Runaway Brain: The Evolution of Human Uniqueness*. New York. Basic Books, A Division of HarperCollins Publishers, Inc.
16. Wells, S. 2003. *The Journey of Man*. New York. Random House Trade Paperbacks.
17. Potter, P.A. & Perry, A.G. 2007. "Spiritual Health". *In Basic Nursing: Essentials for Practice*. (6th ed.) St. Louis, Missouri. Mosby Elsevier.
18. Wills, C. 1993. *The Runaway Brain*, p. 8

DIAGRAM 3.1 THE BEHAVIOR PYRAMID

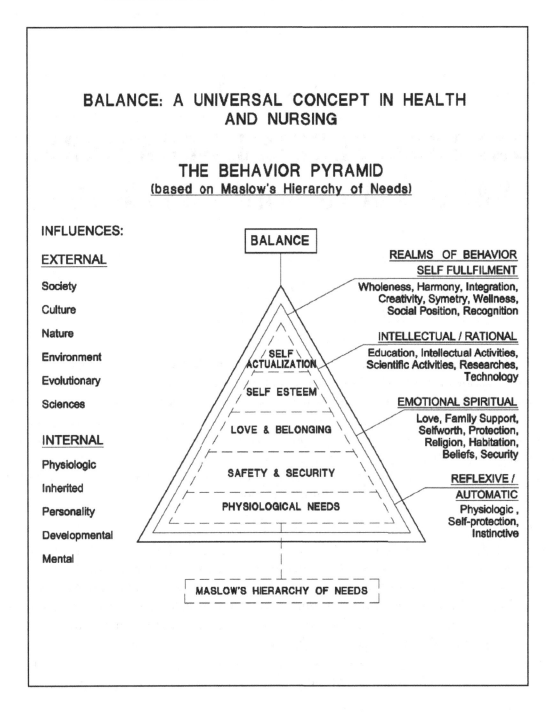

Chapter 4

BALANCE-SEEKING BEHAVIORS: SUBSETS AND MANIFESTATIONS

*"So divinely is the world organized that every one of us, in our
place and time, is in balance with everything else."*
—Adam Acone

The basic premise of this chapter is that balance-seeking is the driver of human behavior, whether consciously or subconsciously, in response to stimuli from the internal and external environment to meet physical, physiological, and psychological needs. These are actions carried out by an individual to satisfy unmet needs. Human behaviors are observable, measurable and describable. Some of these are automatic and instinctive, while others are deliberate. Balance-seeking, as the underlying energy in basic human behavior, is demonstrable through actions that are observable, measurable and describable. Balance—seeking is what separates us human beings from other living beings in the animal kingdom.

Although there are animal behaviors that are quite similar to some human behaviors, these are only observed in some instinctive, or reflexive behaviors that nature has endowed animals to ensure their basic survival. Certain animal behaviors, such as nest building among birds, or squirrels burrowing holes in the ground, are instincts to protect themselves and their young. Maternal instincts in animals to nurse their young have similar behaviors in humans. Migratory patterns of birds are instinctive behaviors. Because lower forms of animals don't have the higher intellectual capacity that humans possess, more complex forms of behavior cannot be observed. This is the greatest advantage of modern humans that enabled the human species to master the planet and explore space that no animals can ever possibly do.

Basic physiologic needs are underlying commonalities among all human beings which are necessary for their physical survival. A newborn has the same need for air, water, food, elimination, and safety as any other individual. It depends on these basic elements for survival. But as the baby grows and matures, other needs emerge, such as its need for love and self-esteem. Psychosocial needs emerge beyond the physiologic. Maturational factors influence their psychosocial needs as they develop their bodies and their minds. The lower physiologic needs will always be present, but other influences determine their psychological needs. Evidence of balance-seeking in both the physiological and psychological realms will become even more evident as the individual matures.

THE BEHAVIOR PYRAMID: REALMS OF HUMAN BEHAVIOR

As previously discussed, balance-seeking behaviors underlie all the realms In the Behavior Pyramid (see Diagram: Behavior Pyramid). The realms of behavior are divided into four categories: 1) reflexive or automatic, 2) emotional/spiritual, 3) intellectual/rational, and 4) Self-fulfillment /Balanced.

As described in the previous chapter, these realms are further reviewed and discussed:

The reflexive or automatic realm is the first and basic level. It includes the basic human needs necessary for physical survival such as air, water, food, elimination, temperature, procreation, sleep and rest. Reflexive behaviors are performed without deliberative thought, such as withdrawing a finger from a flame, or the act of breathing. Other behaviors are instinctive, such as finding water and food because of a natural instinct to eat and drink. Extremes of heat and cold are avoided because of the homeostatic mechanisms in the body that enable the physical body to regulate a stable internal temperature within a normal range. Procreation in lower animals has been a largely instinctive behavior to self-propagate and ensure the survival of the species. As man evolved into a highly sophisticated mammal, sexual behaviors have been regulated by the mores of the culture that ultimately developed. Safety and security needs are also included in this realm. Without safety, the life of the person is endangered. Security is related to the sense of safety on the psychological level. A person who is in a relatively safe and stable building may not necessary feel secure due to other concerns. These concerns are psychological and do not necessarily be related to reality. The roots of lack of security may be tied up with socio-economic concerns, physical threats like bomb and earthquake, or threats to one's freedom.

The emotional /spiritual realm is where more psychosocial needs emerge once the basic physical survival needs are met. Emotions influence human behaviors more as persons experience increasing stimuli from outside environments. Interrelationships in the person's expanding outside world become more important. This realm starts as need for love and affection in the nuclear and extended family and find validation in their relationships with other people outside their immediate sphere of family life. They begin to crave for a sense of belonging to other social groups and to feel like they are part of it. As a sense of belonging is developed, so do the need for self-esteem validation. People who do not find validation of their worth as a person could suffer loss of self—esteem. Personality becomes more and more defined based on their inherited traits, developmental stage, and emotional make-up. Environmental factors, socio-economic status, and family dynamics play a role in shaping personality. Spirituality, as part of culture, starts to develop in this realm. Compassion and caring for others is part of making them feel a sense of belonging and an extension of their feeling of self-worth.

The intellectual/rational realm is a stage entered into by a fully developed, intellectually mature individual who is able to find rationality in their behavior and have developed a realistic perception of the environment. This person sees reality through the lens of their intellect and reason, able to separate irrationality from reason and make judgments based on facts, not emotions. People in this realm find more satisfaction in intellectual and creative pursuits. They seek knowledge for knowledge's sake and use information in ways that benefit them. They make choices based on facts and information. Emotional choices may not necessarily be acceptable to them. As individuals accumulate life experiences going through the previous realms of behavior, the intellectual realm becomes a more satisfying stage. Human development is becoming more complete as the intellectual and emotional realms become more balanced and achieved.

The Self-fulfillment and balance realm is the ultimate stage of balance-seeking human behavior. This is similar to Abraham Maslow's Self-Actualization level where individuals achieve their full potentials. In this realm of behavior, individuals are in a state of optimum physical and mental well-being after having reached and mastered the previous levels. These individuals have obtained, not necessarily success judged from society's standards, but a sense of inner balance and well-being that only comes with a feeling of being loved by others and loving them back, from being respected and respecting others, from knowing the limits of their knowledge and accepting themselves for their limitations, from finding harmony and beauty in the world around them, from respecting and taking good care of their bodies through healthy behaviors, through finding the righteousness and goodness in helping others and accepting help from others, and recognizing that he is but a tiny blip in the timeless movements of the universe. This is the realm of wholeness, the integration of the mind, body and spirit—the ultimate of balance.

Modern thought on human behaviors describes it as performed within systems that consist of inputs, processing, and outputs. A system is a framework within which behavior is performed. As originally proposed by Bertalanffy, Systems Theory was of the view that systems are open to, and interact with their environments.[1] The elements within the system are arranged and related to each other to produce an integrated whole. The system that responds to external forces by eventually returning to their starting points are considered homeostatic.[2] Living systems exhibit homeostatic characteristics in that it is capable of internally correcting itself. By adjusting to the changes produced by either an internal or external stimuli, the organism is able to go back to a stable state or state of balance.

A **holistic** view considers the system as an integrated whole.[3] It emphasizes that the state of the system must be viewed in its entirety and not by its independent parts or elements. It emphasizes that understanding parts of the system will contribute to understanding the whole. This approach is now beginning to be integrated into modern practices in healthcare, management, operations, and the IT industry. Understanding the larger system as well as the contribution of the individual parts to the whole system is key. The holistic approach is important to understanding balance-seeking behaviors. Human balance-seeking behavior does not exist in isolation—it is a product of the dynamic interaction of the internal and external forces processed internally by the human being through its component anatomic structures and functions. Behavior is a manifestation of complex processes influenced by numerous factors both inside and outside of the body.

Human behavior is multi-layered and multi-faceted. Behavior is observable, measurable and describable. Similarly, balance-seeking behavior can be measured, observed and described through its manifestations. Because behavior is so complex, it could be better understood by looking at its subsets or layers, the underlying systems within which it operate, and some general manifestations. These manifestations are demonstrated in at least five subsets of behavior, namely:

- Adaptive
- Physiologic
- Wellness
- Psychosocial
- Physical

ADAPTIVE BEHAVIORS

As described earlier, adaptation is the ability of living organisms to modify themselves over time to take advantage of their environment in order for them to continue to survive. It is said that man is the most successful of animals because he has best adapted to survive—from the harsh savannahs of the African desert to the frozen tundra of the Arctic regions.[4] It is this capacity to adapt to life in any environment that has ensured the survival and success of the human species. Evolutionary processes that happened over vast periods of time and many generations of mankind have produced an animal being that is so different from any other. According to leading geneticist and explorer Spencer Wells, man is biologically adapted to adapt.[5] However, our complex physical adaptive changes did not happen as rapidly as that of lower forms of animals.

Our adaptations came in the form of behavioral changes due to our highly developed brain. The brain, that receives sensory input from the outside environment and chemical signals from within his body, was able to process these stimuli and respond accordingly in terms of adaptive behaviors. The external layer of the skin has largely provided protection for the more delicate internal layers and organs of the body to ensure its integrity and wholeness. Homeostatic mechanisms have allowed continuous monitoring of the internal environment to maintain its chemical and fluid balances. Behaviors of modern human beings have evolved over time and gave rise to complex cultures, language, organizations, technologies, and a wealth of accumulated knowledge that have grown exponentially.

Adaptive behaviors are also responses to changes in the elements of nature that affect all living beings on earth. The balance of nature enabled living beings to survive. Notwithstanding the horrific natural forces that killed large numbers of living things on the face of the earth, such as earthquakes, hurricanes, volcanic eruptions, tsunamis, tornados, etc., human beings managed to survive. After the chaos of cataclysmic events, the earth seems to always go back to a state of stability that continues to promote and support life on this planet. Is this the concept of balance at work?

Recent findings by scientists Kevin Campbell, professor of environmental and evolutionary physiology at the University of Manitoba in Canada and Michael Hofreiter, professor of biology at the University of York in England,[6] and others, revealed how the wooly mammoths, ancient creatures that roamed the earth about two million years ago, were able to adapt to the extreme cold of the environment during the Pliestocene ice ages through physiological processes that made them survive the harsh environment. This adaption of the wooly mammoths did not just alter their physical characteristics but also changed their biochemical adaptations that enabled them to withstand the brutal conditions of the Ice Age world by studying the preserved DNA of these ancient beasts. Much is yet to be revealed in the area of paleophysiology, a new scientific discipline engaged in the study of how the bodies of ancient organisms from the millions of years ago functioned while alive. It might reveal man's fascinating history of adaptation and survival of the human race and how it has evolved to dominate this planet. Evolutionary adaptive changes continue as time goes on, imperceptively perhaps, but only revealed by man's continuous march into history.

PHYSIOLOGIC BEHAVIORS

Physiologic balance-seeking behaviors are not easily observed in real time. However, evidences of physiologic behavior can be measured and inferred through direct observations and laboratory assessments. Underlying physiologic systems include the following: 1. Life support systems, 2. Homeostatic mechanisms, and 3. Defense mechanisms. These systems support balance-seeking behaviors to ensure physical survival of the body.

Life support Systems

As the name suggests, these are systems that support the basic elements of life. These include internal systems in the body that keep the human organism alive. These systems are the **neurologic, cardiovascular**, **respiratory**, and **digestive** systems. The **neurologic system** needs to stay intact in order to regulate all the basal processes of the body. It houses the centers for respirations, blood pressure, hunger, thirst, and heat regulation. Through exquisitely coordinated systems by the brain centers, the body is able to maintain life. The delicate balance of these systems must be maintained automatically. The most immediate need of the body is oxygen, which enables the cells to release the energy locked up in food materials. Brain cells are particularly sensitive to lack of oxygen. Without this life-giving gas, even for a few minutes, the brain cells will die and will instantly snuff out the life of the organism. It will be like a locomotive that dies in the middle of the road when it runs out of fuel.

The **respiratory system** facilitates exchange of oxygen and carbon dioxide, the by-product of cellular metabolism, in the lungs through neural regulation of the process of breathing. Oxygen, which is present in abundance in the atmosphere, must be present and inhaled via the respiratory tract and brought to the lungs to facilitate gas exchange in the air sacs. Failure of any of these structures and processes will prevent the precious gas from reaching the alveoli where gaseous exchange takes place—oxygen is picked up and carbon dioxide is released. The oxygen is then diffused into the blood stream where it is picked up by the hemoglobin in the red blood corpuscles circulating in the blood stream. The oxygen molecules, now combined with hemoglobin (oxy-hemoglobin), is carried to the different cells of the body that are supplied by the blood stream.

In order for the oxygen and nutrients to reach the cells and remove waste products of metabolism, a transport system is needed. This is the role of the **cardiovascular system,** the transport system composed of the heart, its pump, and the vast network of blood-carrying vessels that reaches every cell in the body. If cells do not receive blood supply, they will soon die. However, the body still has a way of reaching those cells that are in danger of dying by establishing alternate routes, called "collateral circulation" to feed blood into parts that do not get their blood supply the normal way. The heart circulation is an example. Being that it is the most important organ in generating the flow of blood with each heartbeat, it is no small wonder that it is equipped with a back-up circulatory mechanism and the capacity to beat ceaselessly throughout the person's life, regulated by nervous control. Failure of the heart to pump will have immediate dire consequences on the body. The brain will immediately suffer the consequences of deprivation of oxygen and nutrients such as glucose. As the circulation fails, toxic products such as carbon dioxide produced by cellular metabolism accumulate. The energy required for the breakdown of nutrients to keep life going rapidly dissipates, and fire of life of the organism is extinguished.

Other life-sustaining elements of the body come from the food and fluids human beings ingest via their **digestive system**. Although the consequences for life are not as immediate as oxygen and circulation, prolonged lack of nutrients and fluids like water, will deprive the cells of the vital elements they need to carry on their work of sustaining life. Fluids and electrolytes, those elements that are present in minute quantities in the body play an important part in balancing the internal environment necessary for sustaining life. The breakdown of nutrients is a prerequisite of life. Aided by a complex system that involves other organs such as the liver for storage and release of nutrients when needed, the enzymes produced by the cells, the hormones which help regulate utilization of nutrients, plus the body's own capacity to produce some proteins, vitamins and minerals, all contribute to keep the body in perfect balance. Without the complex interrelationships of these systems, organs and chemicals, no human life can exist. All these processes occur within the human body systems—the organs and structures that support these processes.

Homeostatic Mechanisms

These mechanisms are responsible for maintaining the constancy of the internal environment of the body. It requires that the body monitors internal conditions and respond appropriately when these conditions deviate from their optimal state. The goal of homeostasis is to maintain stability and equilibrium. Although largely controlled via a system of complex biologic mechanisms, behavioral adaptations enable individuals to balance the effects of changes within the body. It allows an organism to function effectively within a wide range of parameters and still maintain balance of the internal environment. For instance, heat regulation is an internally controlled process. Despite extremes in outside temperatures, the human body maintains a normal core body temperature range of between 36° to 38° Centigrade or 96.8° to 100.4° Fahrenheit measured with a thermometer. Body temperature is the difference between the amount of heat produced by body metabolism and the amount of heat lost to the external environment.[7] For body temperature to stay within normal range, a balance between heat production and heat loss must be maintained. The **hypothalamus** in the brain controls body temperature like a thermostat. Behavioral manifestations of attempts of the body to adjust to temperature changes can be observed such as shivering as an involuntary response to generate more heat and equalize body temperature when the environment is cold. During hot weather, people fan themselves or seek shelter in the shade to balance body temperature. This is another example of a balance-seeking behavior.

There are many other examples of homeostatic balance-seeking behavior at the physiologic level. These physiologic behaviors inside the body can be measured using special instruments: One is the control of blood glucose with insulin and glucagon. The human body maintains a relatively constant blood glucose level, except those who have a problem with glucose regulation controlled by the pancreas. Blood glucose measurements are easily done using glucose monitoring devices. Deviations from normal produce symptoms of either hypoglycemia or hyperglycemia can also be observed through the assessment process. The body has to maintain that delicate balance between too much glucose and too little. Homeostatic mechanisms with its complex system of chemical regulations enable the body to do just that. The act of breathing for example, is automatically triggered in response to sensory mechanisms sensitive to levels of carbon dioxide and oxygen in the blood stream. It can be said that physiologic homeostatic mechanisms exist in order to keep the fire of life burning. The fact that a human being is alive is proof that the body's homeostatic mechanisms are operating within normal parameters.

Defense Mechanisms

Part of the physiologic behavior in human beings is its ability to ward off the invasion of foreign materials such as bacteria, viruses, and other pathogens. It is part of the body's defense mechanism to protect itself and maintain its integrity. The body is already home to many types of bacteria that could be potentially harmful if the body fails to ward off these foreign invaders or keep them at a fairly manageable level. The body has an innate ability to protect itself from injury and infection through a highly sophisticated, multilevel system of defense mechanisms.[8] The first line of defense of the body is the skin that covers the entire body structure. Entry of harmful organisms through portals such as the oral cavity, respiratory tract, and the anus are guarded by built-in structures that keep these organisms from having easy access. Internal defense mechanisms of the body are also built in through its **reticuloendothelial system** composed of white blood cells, lymph nodes, spleen, liver, bone marrow and lungs. Not only can the body defend itself but it also has the ability to repair itself through cellular activities. It also can develop adaptive immunity, or acquired immunity, often called the **immune response**. An effective immune system is able to provide permanent or long-term protection against certain organisms. This ability of the body to maintain a balance between its internal integrity and outside threats is one of the most wondrous adaptive and innate characteristic of human beings. Manifestations that the body's defense mechanisms are working well are demonstrated in the body's maintenance of health and intact immune responses.

WELLNESS BEHAVIORS

We live in an era of health-consciousness, where people are more acutely aware of the concept of wellness and health. Modern scientific discoveries have led to improvements in health care and people are living longer. Literatures are replete with information on how to eat better foods, live a healthy lifestyle, seek positive relationships, and promote a general sense of well-being. Health and wellness are generally used in the same context. The World Health Organization defines health as "a state of complete physical, mental, and social well-being and not merely the absence of disease or infirmity".[9]

The concept of **wellness** is integrated with this definition of health. Wellness is viewed as the incorporation of the physical, emotional, mental and spiritual dimensions. Holism, balance, and homeostasis have been the basic tenets of wellness. The National Wellness Institute, founded in 1977, defines wellness as "an active process through which people become aware of, and make choices toward, a more successful existence".[11] It also acknowledges that there might be different views on what wellness encompasses. Through discussions with leaders in the field of health and wellness, they came up with a general agreement that:

- Wellness is a conscious, self-directed and evolving process of achieving full potential.
- Wellness is multi-dimensional and holistic, encompassing lifestyle, mental and spiritual well-being, and the environment.
- Wellness is positive and affirming.

Eight dimensions of wellness are now recognized by the National Wellness Institute: social, spiritual, physical, intellectual, emotional, occupational, cultural, and environmental.

The precepts of wellness include holism, balance, self-responsibility, and positive attitude. To achieve wellness is to achieve a state of well-being that has the effect of creating balance both within the body and its relationship with the external environment. Making healthy choices to achieve well-being is a cornerstone of wellness. Avoidance of risky behaviors and choosing a lifestyle of moderation and balance contribute to wellness. Seeking spiritual, physical, intellectual, and emotional well-being are goals of balance-seeking. Individuals who practice wellness behaviors are best able to achieve their full potentials and gain greater self-actualization.

Health Care Systems

Health and wellness are supported by existing health care systems and cultures of the society where people live. The modern health care system follows the **biomedical model** which is dominated by advanced technology and use of pharmaceutical medications. Most of the care are provided in hospitals which are generally well-organized, hierarchical, and quite costly. Emphasis is on curing disease, prevention of infection, and moving clients out of hospitals as soon as possible. In many parts of the world however, the **traditional health system** exists where emphasis is on healing not just the physical body but also the emotional, social, and spiritual aspects. The physical realm includes the environment. The concepts of spirituality and harmony with nature are closely intertwined with the concepts of health and wellness.[10] This holistic view has not been widely practiced in the United States and most of the Western world which have adopted the biomedical model of care that focuses on the physical body, or parts of the body, and pathology of diseases that cause illnesses. Curing the disease and treatment of symptoms using surgery and medications manufactured by pharmaceutical companies are standard practice.

Health belief systems: Traditional vs. Biomedical model

In recent years, the wellness view incorporating the holistic approach that is more integrative of traditional approach (often termed complementary or alternative treatment modalities) is gaining momentum. More consumers are incorporating some of their cultural beliefs and practices into the biomedical model. In fact, many people from various cultural backgrounds have been doing just that for a long time. The World Health Organization reported in 2008 that in some Asian and African countries, 80% of the population depended on traditional medicine for primary health care.[14] WHO describes Traditional medicine as the sum total of knowledge, skills and practices based on the theories, beliefs and experiences indigenous to different cultures that are used to maintain health, as well as prevent, diagnose, improve or treat physical and mental illness. Herbal treatments are the most widely-used form of traditional medicine. Health care professionals practicing within the modern western health care systems are recognizing the value of **complementary** and **alternative therapies** as part of their care. Nursing, with its holistic approach, has led the way in incorporating some of these practices from its early beginnings. Medical practitioners of the biological model have yet to incorporate the Traditional model in their practice. It seems that as the practice of medicine becomes more and more specialized, the approach to care becomes more compartmentalized. The "wholeness" view appear to become more and more limited under the biomedical model.

Health-seeking Behaviors

Wellness behaviors are health-seeking. A sense of well-being and increased energy level are outcomes of wellness behaviors. **Health-seeking** describes the conscious or subconscious attempt of the individual to find physical and psychosocial balance. Physical and mental equilibrium are manifestations of balance. Physical equilibrium can be achieved through healthy habits such as regular exercise, eating balanced meals, avoiding risky physical activities, and prevention of diseases and infections. Mental equilibrium involves the ability to cope with emotional and mental stresses that constantly inundate modern living. Job-related stresses are known to be sources of mental and emotional imbalance. Social relationships with family members or others in the person's social network also create either positive or negative influences on one's mental equilibrium. A loving, supportive relationship contributes to well-being; a contentious, adversarial relationship is a source of negative feelings.

What is truly amazing about the human body is its ability to repair itself, heal itself, regulate itself, defend itself, and keep its internal environment constant and balanced so that it will continue to maintain life. The moment that these abilities are jeopardized, the body goes into an unbalanced state. When not corrected, it will continue on a downward spiral that will eventually lead to its extinction. Notwithstanding these built-in mechanisms, humans also have the instinct for survival that could defy unbelievable odds. Many patients live to tell their stories of overcoming life-threatening disease conditions. It seems that there are commonalities to their stories of survival: the positive, self-affirming attitude, the striving to overcome their condition, the mental and spiritual well-being, a lifestyle devoted to wellness, and the greater consciousness of their relationship with nature and their environment. These are all elements of wellness that advocates have been trying to promote for increased quality of life and longevity. Optimum health can be achieved within the social and health systems, regardless of philosophy, that emphasizes wellness and health-seeking behaviors.

PSYCHOSOCIAL BEHAVIORS

Psychosocial behaviors encompass a wide area of human behavior. As social beings, humans have developed various systems to achieve their need to interact and live with other humans harmoniously and productively. Early on in its existence, humans appeared to understand the value of living with others—first with their nuclear family, and over time, with others as they expanded and developed communities. It is not clear how structured societies developed from man's early isolated beginnings but it shows that such behaviors were undoubtedly linked to adaptation and self-preservation. The advanced material culture of modern man can be attributed to mental and physical adaptations of their highly developed body and brain that enabled the human species to survive until the present time. It did not just physically thrive; it also developed complicated social, organizational, religious, economic, cultural, and technological systems within which modern man finds the ultimate satisfactions of their basic and higher needs.

Psycho-social behaviors are performed and observed within various underlying systems:

- Personality systems

- Cultural belief systems
- Religious belief systems
- Family systems
- Organizational systems

Personality Systems

A systems approach to personality is described by John Mayer in his book "Personality: A Systems Approach." Personality is defined as "habitual patterns and qualities of behavior expressed by physical and mental activities and attitudes; the distinctive individual qualities of a person."[15] A person's personality is defined by his or her personality traits or qualities that are unique to each person. A social being starts with a person having a personality or self that interacts with others. Different theories on personality view the development of personality in various ways. Behavioral theorists such as B.F. Skinner and John B. Watson believe that personality is influenced by heredity and environment. Biological theorists propose that genetics are responsible for personality. This school of thought suggests the link between genetics and personality traits. Psychodynamic theories such as Sigmund Freud's influence of the unconscious mind and Erik Erikson's stages of psychosocial development attempt to explain the development of personality. Humanist theories that include the works of Carl Rogers and Abraham Maslow emphasize the concept of self-actualization.[16]

But personality is so complex and varies from one person to another. The factors that influence one person may not be the same ones that affect another, even in the same family or community. Behavior involves an interaction between the person's underlying personality and situational or environmental factors. Many researchers believe that there are at least five broad categories of personality trait that are universal such as: extraversion, agreeableness, conscientiousness, neuroticism, and openness.[16] A study of people from more than 50 different cultures found that these broad dimensions of personality could be accurately used to describe personality. Based on this research, it is now believed by many psychologists that the five personality dimensions are not only universal but also have biological origins. These are core personality traits suggested by psychologist David Buss as an evolutionary explanation that shaped social behaviors and relationships over time.[17]

These theories point to the difficulty in identifying the true origins of personality. The basic question is, what determined personality during the early beginnings of the human being and how did it evolve and contribute to their survival over time? If personality was genetically determined according to the biological theorists, what shaped the diversity of human personalities as they continued to survive in their small and simple communities to the more complex ones in modern era? Did man's nature as a social being evolve from this genetically-determined personality, or did personality contribute to the evolution of man as a social being? The answer perhaps lies in the proverbial chicken or the egg dilemma. No one knows for sure.

How does personality play a part in balance-seeking behaviors? I suggest that the five core dimensions of personality identified earlier determine how one is able to achieve balance in their lives. Each of these dimensions represent a continuum between two extremes. A balanced personality represents a middle ground somewhere between. The polar opposite of each trait lies in the domain of imbalance and abnormality. For instance, extraversion is the trait that includes such characteristics as excitability, sociability, talkativeness, assertiveness and high amounts of emotional energy. The opposite is introversion, an inwardly-focused personality and avoids social interaction. This is similar to the trait of openness which is characterized by imagination and insight, and tends to have a broad range of interest. In contrast, a closed personality is narrow-minded, opinionated, and unimaginative.

Personality also determines a person's response to psychological stress. **Coping mechanisms** vary from one person to another as well. These are the psychological mechanisms that allow a person to manage their stress levels in a way that enable a person to achieve a certain sense of balance. Emotional responses are manifested in various behaviors positively or negatively—crying, shouting, laughing, anger, resentment, remorse, elation, joy, sadness, etc. These responses trigger physiologic and psychological reactions which the body will seek to normalize through balance-seeking behaviors. Developmental stages affect the manner in which a person interprets and perceives situations mediated by the person's core personality. For instance, a normally extroverted teen-ager will react with excessive joy to a good news but an introverted personality will react with nonchalance or lack of emotion. Each person's personality will influence the coping mechanism that a person will use to achieve psychological balance. Balance-seeking behaviors will be manifested accordingly.

Cultural Beliefs

Culture is variously defined. One definition by Giger and Davidhizar is that culture as "a patterned behavioral response that develops over time as a result of imprinting the mind through social and religious structures and intellectual and artistic manifestations."[18] Furthermore, they affirm that although culture is a result of acquired mechanisms, it is also affected by internal and external environmental stimuli. Spector acknowledges that there is no single definition of culture but it is learned by people from their environment and a medium of social relationships shared and passed on from one generation to the next[19].

Every culture has its own set of beliefs to which people in that group subscribe. Some of these include beliefs about religion and spirituality, health and illness, healing, values, family relationships and child-rearing, death and dying, food preferences, communication patterns, and rituals. Despite wide differences among cultural groups, there are basic characteristics of culture:[20] 1. culture is learned and taught, 2. culture is shared, 3. culture is social in nature, 4. culture is dynamic, adaptive and ever-changing.

Culture enables individuals and groups to adapt to meet environmental changes. These changes in beliefs and practices within a culture occur slowly or rapidly, depending on the factors that brought the changes. For instance, wars on a large scale, could rapidly change the social and political structure of a culture and dynamically change their core belief systems. Culture is the group's response to its common needs. The dynamic and adaptive nature of culture enables it to survive and gets passed on from one generation to the next. The social nature of culture is consistent with the social nature of human beings. Man has survived throughout history through living with other human beings from birth to death. At times, human beings also cause the extinction of themselves and others. But for the most part, human beings have learned to protect each other and themselves through social organizations. Culture is an essential element of human survival.

Family Systems

That the family is a psychosocial system is an accepted concept in the social sciences and medicine. Systems theory recognizes that the family as a unit utilizes and functions with input from the external environment and society, and influences the behavior of its members. Family dynamics could change individual responses to information obtained from outside its boundaries. It has its own hierarchical organization, relational structure, boundaries, genetic characteristics, and a means by which culture is passed on from one generation to another. It provides the supporting structure which enables family members to find balance and stability while they develop from childhood to maturity. From primitive societies to modern complex ones, the family has served to provide most of its members' needs. It is a universal social institution from which other social institutions such as government, religion, and education have evolved. Families even within the same culture vary in their practices. But certain common beliefs, values, and attitudes are found among families in the same culture.

The family is the basic social structure of society which performs three functions: socialization, affection and companionship, and sexual regulation.[21] Of these, the function of providing affection and companionship provides the most element of balance to its members. Love and affection are among man's most basic psychosocial needs. Esteem needs are met through family support and positive relationships. Inability to find these emotional-psychological elements within the family often results in disorders—an emotional and psychological imbalance. Childhood experiences influence individual personality and determine their ability to cope with future stresses as individuals become mature.

From the biological perspective, the family is the social unit that functions to perpetuate the species through nurturing and protective behaviors of the parents or parent-surrogate towards their young. This behavior has also been observed in the animal kingdom where mothers would fight other predatory animals to protect their young. This maternal instinct has survived in the human species and thus ensured the continued propagation of the species. The predominant family is the nuclear family consisting of parents (or a parent) and their non-adult children living in the same household. Although this concept of the nuclear family in modern society is changing, it is still the basic family unit in most cultures. It provides the framework within which children first learn to relate with others and enable them to develop their own personalities, learn basic human values, assume their roles within the family, and develop skills to interact with the outside world. When adaptive mechanisms are used by the family, internal equilibrium by its members is facilitated. Similarly, when adaptive mechanisms fail, the equilibrium is disturbed and psychological disturbances could result during the child's development.

Organizational systems

The nucleus of human social organizations is the family. Organizations have primary goals, structure and function. According to Giger and Davidhizar, the American culture has two primary goals that are inherent to the family: (1) nurturing and encouragement of its family members and (2) the development of independent and healthy children.[22] The typical family structure is composed of a hierarchy with the parents as the authority figures, and the offspring at various levels in the hierarchy, often depending on their birth order. The function of the family is to provide for basic needs such as food, shelter, safety, love, and belongingness in order for family members to survive and become contributing members of society. These functions are directed towards meeting the primary goals of the family.

As the human race flourished, society became more diverse and more complex organizations emerged—products of the increasingly intelligent, educated, and creative human beings that inhabit the earth. Humans have found a way to increase their ability to survive by creating complicated forms of social organizations and various ways of dividing labor so that each member of society is counted upon to contribute to the greater good of the many. However, some individuals have used power to their advantage, either through physical force, material resources, and ability to mobilize, or sometimes coerce, the cooperation and capacities of others to gain control and influence in society. However, without the balancing effects of those who believe in the concept of equality and social equilibrium, human societies become imbalanced and uneven with advantages stacked up on one side versus both sides.

Along with the development of human societies and organizations were the work stresses and psychosocial problems that are inevitable by-products of human relationships. Roles in society became more defined and yet diverse. Socio-economic conditions have largely influenced the manner in which organizations evolved over time. Social issues such as justice, equality, power, morality, wealth distribution, racial discrimination, marriage, and gender roles may occupy center stage at some point in time. The search for more wealth and economic power has become a strong motivation for many people. Seeking balance of these issues in one's personal life becomes a major challenge. These are potential sources of psychological stress which could affect individuals. Stress causes psychological and physical imbalances, as discussed in previous parts of the book. To find balance, adaptive mechanisms must be adopted by the individual. Balance-seeking could be in the form of obtaining professional help from a psychiatrist or psychologist, practicing healthy lifestyles, exercise, good nutrition and avoiding risky behaviors.

Religious belief systems

Religion is widely recognized as an institution found in all societies. It is not easy to define precisely because the term describes behavior that vary widely from culture to culture and from individual to individual. It has sacred and spiritual aspects but, according to sociologists, it is also shaped by the culture and environment of each society. There are various definitions of religion, including Webster dictionary's narrow definition that religion is a "belief in and worship of God or gods; or a specific system of belief, worship, etc., often involving a code of ethics."[23] There are two components of religion that must be distinguished from one another according to Popenoe:[24] one, the universal human impulse toward religion, with its spiritual basis; and two, the social form in which it is expressed and institutionalized.

It is not clear how religion began, whether the universal impulse for the divine and a sacred power was an impetus to establish religious institutions. Or it could be the inherent spiritual nature of man that inexplicably led to belief in a higher power greater than themselves. Perhaps, it is also a means for man to relinquish control of his destiny to one that is more powerful and all-knowing. Or perhaps, it is rooted in the vulnerability of man and the search for that stability in his life that only a powerful god or spirit can provide. One commonality among religions is the idea of the **sacred**—be it an object, a place, a person, or an intangible being that evokes special respect and reverence. It could also evoke feelings of fear and dread if the person does not follow the codes of behavior that the religion dictates. Ancients have worshiped objects in nature and practiced their religious rituals to preserve what they considered as sacred.

Organized religions are practiced within social systems that meets basic psychological needs and provide a sense of stability to those who experience some fundamental problems in human existence. In man's search for balance and harmony, religion has provided the psychological underpinning and guiding philosophy in how individuals can live their lives. The principle of balancing opposites in order to find the **"center"**—the place where opposites balance each other and be in a state of harmony, has long been practiced in cultures around the world, especially the eastern world. This polarity of opposites also highlights the importance of finding inner balance and harmony. It can be inferred that since the beginning of human existence, man has possessed the need for balancing the opposites in their lives. Throughout the ages, man has experienced conditions of extremes—nature, emotions, lifestyles, economic conditions, etc. Their religious beliefs and spirituality probably provided them with the emotional strength to find their inner balance and harmony, thus enabling them to weather life's stresses. This concept of balance found its way in many cultural beliefs and practices around the world and has endured through centuries of human existence.

PHYSICAL BEHAVIOR: MUSCULOSKELETAL SYSTEMS AND EMOTIONAL BEHAVIOR

Most of behavioral manifestations are observed through physical actions apparent to others. But these actions reflect the amazing coordination of all the internal structures inside the body of a human being—from the approximately 206 bones in the adult skeleton, to the joints, muscles, tendons, and connective tissues that work together to form the physical structure of every single person. Even more amazing is the fact that some of these structures can work automatically without conscious effort, such as the heart muscles, the smooth muscles of the gastrointestinal tract, the smooth muscles of the walls of blood vessels, and other organs like the urinary bladder and the eyes. It is an integrated open system that receives input or stimuli from its environment, has the ability to process complicated data and information at lightning speed, and produces outputs in terms of behavior.

The human body is built to correct and maintain itself through a system of voluntary and involuntary muscles—those that can be consciously controlled and those that work automatically to maintain basic functions. Those basic functions are aimed to maintain life at the most primal level—maintenance of heart beat, blood pressure, breathing, nutrition, and elimination. However, it is still the central command center that exerts control over all body functions—the brain. Without this central control center, life cannot continue as it was designed to exist. Modern science has tried to mimic the functions of these organs with some degree of success—the artificial heart, the mechanical ventilators, the digestive aids, etc. However, these devices have failed to function the way human organs do. No one has yet invented a machine that performs the same level exquisitely found in human beings.

The skeleton acts as the internal scaffolding that compose the physical structure of the human body. In order for the body to maintain its physical balance and walk upright, it needs to have an intact brain that can control movement and process information fed to it by the senses. Man has been endowed by nature with the ability to perform movements—from physical skills such as running, jumping, and climbing, to delicate and intricate movements such as threading a needle or repairing a watch. The motor cortex is the main center for the planning, initiation, and execution of all body movements.

Physical behavior alone is not just a mechanical manifestation of the body's actions. It also reflects emotions that give clues to the inner feelings of the individual. Emotions are often the universal language of the soul but could also be modified by cultural practices. For instance, crying is a universal expression of sadness; it could also express happiness. Anger manifestations are universally expressed as aggressive and destructive behavior, but it could also be manifested as crying. Laughing generally indicates happiness but it could also denote derision and contempt to some. Emotional behavior therefore may not necessarily be a good physical indicator of the inner emotional state of the person.

How physical behavior can contribute to balance-seeking is in finding a congruence between body and spirit. It is obvious that there is a need to first maintain physical health to achieve a sense of balance and well-being. A sense of well-being starts with a healthy body, free of disease and disability. Well-being manifests itself in being able to care for oneself, seek fulfillment of one's personal goals, and meeting needs. Lack of well-being eventually contributes to physical and emotional imbalance, leading to illness and death if not corrected. Maintaining physical balance can be as simple as getting adequate rest and sleep. Exercise can strengthen muscles, bones, and physical stamina to withstand environmental stresses. Good nutrition and healthy food choices contribute to physical health and well-being. The adage "you are what you eat" has proven true in many ways. Minimizing stresses contributes to physical health and well-being.

KEY CONCEPTS

1. Balance-seeking behaviors are demonstrated by all human beings—a common denom—inator of the human race. It is driven by stimuli from the internal and external environment to meet physiological, physical, and psychological needs to ensure self-preservation and achieve self-fulfillment. These behaviors are observable, measurable and describable.
2. Balance-seeking behaviors underlie all the realms in the Behavior Pyramid which are divided into four categories based on Maslow's Hierarchy of Needs Pyramid: 1. Reflexive or automatic realm, 2) Emotional/Spiritual realm, 3) Intellectual/Rational realm, 4) Self-fulfillment and Balance realm.
3. Human behavior is multi-layered and multi-faceted. Balance-seeking is an aspect of human behavior whose manifestations can be demonstrated and observed in

at least five sub-sets of behavior, namely: 1) Adaptive, 2) Physiologic, 3) Wellness, 4) Psychosocial, and 5) Physical. The complexity of human behavior can be better understood by looking at these subsets and the underlying systems within which each operates.

4. Adaptive behavior springs from the capacity for adaptation characteristic of living beings to modify themselves over time in order to survive changes in their environment. Human adaptation took the form of both physical and psychological changes due to its highly developed brain. Biological and physical adjustments in response to external factors enabled human beings as well as other animals on the planet to survive.

5. Manifestations of physiologic behavior can best be measured through instruments and inferred through observations. Underlying physiologic systems such as life support systems, homeostatic mechanisms, and internal defense mechanisms support balance-seeking behaviors to ensure physical survival of the body.

6. Wellness behaviors encompass the balance of the physical, emotional, mental and spiritual dimensions—a holistic approach. Balance is achieved through the precepts of health and wellness—concepts that are intimately intertwined. Eight dimensions of wellness are recognized by the National Wellness Institute. Individuals who practice wellness behaviors are best able to achieve their full potentials and gain greater level of self-fulfillment.

7. Health and wellness are supported by health care systems and the cultures where people live. There are two basic health belief systems that exist: Traditional and Biomedical models. Each has its own set of beliefs, practices, and institutions: the Biological model emphasizes curing diseases through pharmaceutical and scientific modalities; the Traditional or alternative treatment modalities focus on healing by incorporating cultural practices and herbal treatments passed on through generations.

8. Psychosocial behaviors encompass a wide range of human behavior that defines man as a social being. The need to live with and interact with other human beings was perhaps born, not just out of the necessity for survival, but also the need for human relationships. I appears that even in the beginning of its existence as a social animal, man apparently understood the value of living with others—first with the nuclear family and then with others in the community. Over time, social groups expanded to form structured organizations and societies to the complex institutions we see today.

9. Psychosocial behaviors developed within various underlying systems: personality system, family systems, cultural belief systems, religious belief systems, organizational systems, and creative/technological systems. Paradoxically, while these systems create imbalances in human existence through the stresses complex societies produce, these also enable man to find psychosocial balance and stability when dealt with positively.

10. Physical behaviors are outward manifestations of the state of the body that are directly observable. Although not always obvious, it is also a reflection of the emotional status

and feeling states of the individual. Human actions reflect the coordination of all the internal structures of the body regulated by the centers in the brain. The human body is an integrated system affected by, and responds to, stimuli from the environment. The balance of the physical body and emotional states contributes to the overall well-being of the individual.

CHAPTER 4: BALANCE-SEEKING BEHAVIORS: SUBSETS AND MANIFESTATIONS

REFERENCES

1. Heylighen, F. and Joslyn, C. 1992. *What is Systems Theory?* (Prepared for the Cambridge Dictionary of Philosophy). http://pespmc1.vub.ac.be/SYSTHEOR.html. retrieved 4/14/2012.

2. Systems Theory/Order-Chaos-Wikibooks, *Openbooks for an open world*. http://en.wikibooks. org/wiki/Systems_Theory/Order-Chaos.retrieved 4/14/2012.

3. Systems Theory/Holism-Wikibooks, *Open books for an open world*. http://en.wikibooks.org/ wikiSystems_Theory/Holism. retrieved 4/14/2012.

4. McNally, Rand & Company. 1980. *Funk & Wagnalls: Atlas of the Body and Mind*. Illinois. Mitchell Beazley Publishers.

5. Wells, S. 2002. *The Journey of Man*. Princeton, N.J. Princeton University Press, p. 89.

6. Campbell, K. and Hofreiter, M. August, 2012. "A New life for Ancient DNA", in *Scientific American*, 307 (2), 46-51.

7. Potter, A.P. and Perry, A.G. 2005. *Fundamentals of Nursing* (6th ed.) St. Louis, Missouri. Mosby, Inc./Elsevier Inc.

8. Huether, S.E. and McCance, K.L. 2008. *Understanding Pathophysiology* (4th ed.) St. Louis, Missouri. Mosby, Inc. /Elsevier, Inc.

9. Preamble to the Constitution of the World Health Organization as adopted by the International Health Conference, New York, 19-22 June, 1946; signed on 22 July 1946 by the representatives of the 61 States (Official Records of the World Health Organization, no.2, p.100) and entered into force on 7 April 1948. The definition has not been amended since 1948.

10. Lewis, et al. 2007. *Medical-Surgical Nursing*. St. Louis, Missouri. Mosby, 94-109.

11. National Wellness Institute. Defining wellness. http://www.nationalwellness.org/index.php. retrieved 9/04/2012.

12. Guralnik, D.B. (Ed). 1982. *Webster's New World Dictionary of the American Language*. New York. Simon & Schuster.

13. Mayer, J. D. 1998. A systems framework for the field of personality psychology. *Psychological Inquiry*, *9*, 118-144.

14. World Health Organization Fact Sheet. Dec. 2008. *Traditional Medicine*. http://www.who. int/mediacentre/factsheets/fs134/en/. Retrieved 9/04/2012.

15. Frisch, N.C. & Frisch, L.E. 2002. *Psychiatric Mental Health Nursing—Understanding the Client as well as the Condition* (2ⁿᵈ ed.) New York. Delmar.

16. Cherry, K. *The Big five personality dimensions: 5 major factors of personality.* http://psychology.about.com/od/personality development/a/bigfive.html. retrieved 9/13/2012.

17. Buss, D.M. 1995. "Evolutionary Psychology: a New Paradigm for Psychological Science". *Psychological Inquiry.* p.1-31.

18. Giger,J.N. and Davidhizar,R.E. 1995. *Transcultural Nursing* (2ⁿᵈ ed.)St. Louis, Missouri. Mosby.

19. Spector, R.E. 2009. *Cultural Diversity in Health and Illness* (7ᵗʰ ed.) New Jersey. Prentice Hall. p.9-11.

20. Daniels, R. 2004. *Nursing Fundamentals: Caring & Clinical Decision Making.* New York. Delmar, p. 91-112.

21. Popenoe, D. 1977. *Sociology* (3ʳᵈ ed.) Englewood Cliff, New Jersey Prentice-Hall, Inc., p.185-188.

22. Giger, J.N. and Davidhizar, R.E. 1995. *Transcultural Nursing* (2ⁿᵈ ed.) St. Louis, Missouri. Mosby. P.70

23. Agnes, M. (Ed.) 2002. Webster's *New Dictionary and Thesaurus.* Cleveland, Ohio. Wiley Publishing, Inc.

24. Popenoe, D. 1977. *Sociology* (3ʳᵈ ed.) p. 366-367.

TABLE 4.1: BALANCE-SEEKING BEHAVIORS:
SUBSETS AND MANIFESTATIONS

SUB-SETS OF BEHAVIORS	UNDERLYING SYSTEMS	SOME GENERAL MANIFESTATIONS
ADAPTIVE	Evolutionary process Ecological systems	Physical adaptive changes over time Balance of nature
PHYSIOLOGIC	Life Support Systems Homeostatic Mechanisms Defense Mechanisms	Basal life indicators Basic needs fulfillment Physiologic indicators Immune system intact
WELLNESS	Health Care System Health Belief Systems (Western vs. Traditional)	Health-seeking behaviors Well-being, energy level Physical and mental equilibrium
PSYCHO-SOCIAL	Personality Systems Socio-economic systems Cultural belief systems Family Systems Organizational Systems Religious belief systems Technological/creative systems	Coping mechanisms to stress Emotional responses Developmental stages Income-production, business behaviors Norms, values, cultural practices Family roles and relationships Roles in society; sense of justice & equality

		Spirituality, Harmony with God and nature
		Scientific, Symmetry, Artistry, Musicality
PHYSICAL	Physical body system	Physical fitness and development
	Environmental elements	Safety, stability, and protection from elements
	Structural systems	

Chapter 5

BALANCE AND CULTURE

"One of the results of having a highly adaptive mind is the development of the complex culture".
—Spencer Wells, The Journey of Man

"A nation's culture resides in the hearts and in the souls of its people"
—Mahatma Gandhi

It is not the purpose of this chapter to explore the origins of culture. This would be purely conjecture without solid research evidence of how culture developed. But scientists like Spencer Wells in his "Journey of Man"[1] ascribed the development of culture to man's extraordinarily superior brain and social interactions. It is complex culture that is unique to the human species and makes us what we are today—a product of adaptive, evolutionary process dependent on balancing forces for survival. Culture influences behavior and all aspects of life, including attitudes, beliefs and values.[2]

BALANCE CONCEPTS IN CULTURE

Culture is defined by various authors.[3,4,5,6,7] Giger and Davidhizar define it as a patterned response that develops over time imprinted through social and religious structures and artistic manifestations. Leininger, Spector, Boyle & Andrews, and Purnell & Paulanka have various definitions of culture. There is so much diversity among cultural groups but there are characteristics that are common denominators basic to all cultures. These characteristics are identified as:[2] 1) Culture is learned and taught, 2) Culture is shared, 3) Culture is social in nature, 4) Culture is dynamic, adaptive and ever-changing. Cultural beliefs, values, customs, and behaviors are transmitted from one generation to another.

The enduring elements of culture have left footprints for the next generations to follow and pass on to the next. The elements of health care beliefs and healing practices have withstood the changes in values over time. It is most important to note for the purposes of this book that BALANCE is a concept that is found in most cultures around the world. It probably has a direct relationship with the human tendency for the body systems to interact and maintain a constant physiological state called homeostasis mentioned earlier in the book as an element of survival.

Health and Illness Concepts—Allopathic vs. Homeopathic

The balance concept is the foundation of many health-illness and spiritual beliefs in most cultures around the world. Health is perceived as a state of balance; illness is a state of imbalance. There is a universal prevailing belief within most traditional cultures that a person must be in a state of balance with the family, community, and the forces of the natural world around him or her. Or, one might be in a state of imbalance with the family, the community, or the forces of the natural world in one or all aspects of the person. Health is achieved through balance or harmony of the mind and body using different traditional methods of maintenance, protection, and restoration. A holistic philosophy guides these traditional practices in that all facets of a person are considered: physical, mental, and spiritual. In this traditional context, health has interrelated facets, represented by: 1) health maintenance, 2) health protection, and 3) health restoration.

It is necessary to revisit the concepts of health and illness and explore their meanings in terms of the role of balance. Spector defines health as "the balance of the person, both within one's beings—physical, mental, and spiritual—and in the outside world—natural, communal, and metaphysical, is a complex, interrelated phenomenon ". Illness on the other hand, is "the imbalance of one's being—physical, mental and spiritual—and in the outside world—natural, communal and metaphysical"[8]. Health/Illness and balance are closely intertwined: health cannot exist without balance; lack of balance results in illness. Health is viewed from a holistic standpoint—a balance of all aspects of the human body—physical, mental and spiritual. But health philosophies of modern Western societies subscribe to the **allopathic** model adopted by the American Medical Association. It only accepts modalities that are proven by scientific methods and empirical evidences in the treatment of diseases. Allopathic health care does not take into consideration traditional healers and providers of health care such as herbalists, osteopaths, homeopaths, chiropractors, medicine men and women—people what have provided health care to ill members of the community through methods that have been accepted in the culture of that group of people. On the other hand, **homeopathic** philosophy treats the person, not just the disease and espouses a holistic approach. It is the philosophy that sees health as a balance of the physical, mental and spiritual whole. The difference between these two philosophies lays bare the divergence of philosophies in dealing with health and illness.

Homeopathic care actually encompasses a wide range of health care practices that are not practiced by allopathic medicine. These are often referred to as "complementary medicine" or "alternative medicine". **Complementary medicine** is further broken down into two categories: 1) alternative or integrative, and 2) traditional or ethnocultural. Alternative therapies such as aromatherapy, acupuncture, biofeedback, hypnotherapy, massage therapy, and reflexology, are those that are generally not part of one's ethnocultural or religious heritage. Traditional therapies such as *ayurvedic and curanderismo,* are part of one's traditional ethnocultural or religious heritage. Although the *Qi gong, reiki, Santeria, and voodoo* therapies do not conform to the standards set by the allopathic medical community, the attitude and acceptance by many members of the community are changing. The holistic approach is gradually being integrated into medical practice. Nursing has long practiced the holistic approach in caring for patients since the advent of modern nursing. It is this holistic view of health and illness that appears to be more compatible with the wholeness of human beings and a culturally appropriate approach.

Whether health is approached from the allopathic or the homeopathic standpoints, the common ground in these philosophies is that health is a state of balance that must be maintained, protected, and restored. Health beliefs and practices may change over time as people's experiences change. But traditional methods of health maintenance, protection, and restoration have withstood the test of time and have been passed on from generation to generation. Some practices may have been debunked by modern scientific evidences. But the enduring and underlying view of health as a state of balance has persisted throughout history.

The Mind-Body connection: Chi, Yin and Yang

Some cultures, particularly the Asian cultures, define physiological balance in terms of an energy called **chi.**[9] The balance of chi creates harmony between the mind and the body and maintains overall health. In this view, the mind-body connection is the cornerstone of health and wellness.

Harmony of mind and body is embodied in the balance between the forces of the **yin** and **yang** in the traditional Chinese wellness belief. Yin and yang represent opposing and complementary aspects of the universal energy chi present within the human body. According to the Chinese view, the goal in a healthy life is to maintain a harmonious balance between yin and yang forces. Yang forces are characterized as light, positive, creative, energetic, and having the nature of heaven. Yin forces are characterized as dark, negative, quiet, receptive and having the nature of earth. These two opposing forces are also complementary aspects of chi.

This Asian philosophy of the mind-body connection are inseparable. Balancing the yin and yang forces creates a state of harmony of the whole person and restores and promotes health. A state of harmony is a state of equilibrium where opposing forces balance each other. This impulse to seek balance is nature's way to enable human beings to survive by adapting to their internal and external environments. This is achieved through a highly developed brain that controls human behavior, emotions and feelings. It is the springboard of all human activities.

The mind-body connection is an important element of culture discovered and practiced by people since the ancient times. It has found its way in many aspects of life with infinite variations from culture to culture—health and illness beliefs, spiritual and religious practices, interpersonal relationships, food practices, activities of daily living, birth and death rituals, etc. Homeostatic mechanisms provide the impetus for many of man's behaviors to seek fulfillment of needs. These are influenced by signals from the brain that affect physiological functions and emotional responses. Disturbances in centers in the brain that processes these signals, as well as those centers in the brain responsible for thoughts and feelings, can disrupt the normal activities of the nervous, endocrine, and immune systems. These are functions of the human body that need to be balanced in order to maintain health and wellness, and ultimately, its survival. Cultural practices are behaviors that are derived from patterned responses to maintain balance in everyday life—from beliefs in a higher power of a god or nature to maintain emotional strength and stability, to eating foods that sustain life and health and keep the body in balance, to healing practices through the use of traditional remedies, to the use of symbolic objects to protect health. These, and numerous other practices, are parts of culture of a given group of people that are passed on from generation to generation throughout the ages.

BALANCE BELIEFS IN CULTURES AROUND THE WORLD

In many cultures around the world, the balance concept is related to health and illness beliefs, which also extend to other practices in their daily lives affecting their health. This belief is imbedded in many aspects of life and health—through balance in temperatures, food, child-rearing, childbirth, medicines, healing, spiritual health, and supernatural beliefs. Typically, health is viewed as being in harmony with nature; illness is a state of disharmony. Related concepts of balance such as harmony, symmetry, stability, equality, and well-being pervade all areas of life in cultures around the world. Balance is interwoven in the basic fabric of human life. All the cultures of the world can be viewed as a universal tapestry with balance as the common thread. Health practices differ widely from one culture to another but the concept of balance in health appears to be a commonality. By examining some traditional cultural practices of health maintenance, health protection, and health restoration among various groups of peoples, this common theme emerges.

In the book **Culture and Clinical Care**,[10] most of the thirty-five different cultures featured in the book mentioned balance or concepts of balance as part of their cultural beliefs, particularly related to health and illness beliefs. The authors of each chapter belong to the specific cultural group described and have intimate knowledge of the culture to which they belong. The following are direct quotes from chapter authors from each cultural group (elements of balance and related concepts are bolded):

1. Afghans (Juliene Lipson and Razia Askaryar): Illness can have natural causes such as "germs", dirt, cold or wind, seasonal changes, or not taking proper care of one's body. A traditional humoral belief is that "hot" and "cold" **imbalances** cause sickness; hot/cold qualities describe food, drinks, medicinal herbs, individual human nature, and specific illnesses.
2. African Americans (Catherine Waters and Salamah Locks): Typically view health as being in **harmony** with nature and illness as a state of **disharmony.**
3. American Indians/Alaskan Natives (Janelle Palacios, Rose Butterfly, and C. June Strickland): Some AI/AN relate physical illness to violation of taboos or being out of **harmony,** although beliefs may vary depending on culture, assimilation and individuals beliefs.
4. Arabs (Afaf Ibrahim Meleis): Naturalistic and social causes of illness include bad luck, stress in the family, loss of person or objects, "germs", winds and drafts, **imbalance** in hot/cold and dry/mist, and sudden fears.
5. Cambodians (Judith Kulig and Sanom Prak): Many attribute illness to natural or supernatural causes. Natural causes include **imbalance** in "hot"/"cold" or other forces.
6. Central Americans—Guatemalans, Nicaraguans, and Salvadorans (Paul Kunkel, Damaris Aragon, and Mirna Meono de Kunkel): Ill health results from **imbalance**, thus the concern about "hot"/"cold" and strong/weak.
7. Chinese (Pauline Chin): Consider food important for maintaining body's **balance** of "cold" (yin) and "hot" (yang). Believe that yin-yang **imbalance** causes illness.
8. East Indians (Rachel Zachariah): Ayurvedic philosophy attributes illness to an **imbalance** in body humors, which creates circulating toxins that accumulate in weaker areas of body.
9. Ethiopians and Eritreans (Yewoubdar Beyene): Concept of health: A state of **equilibrium** among physiological, spiritual, cosmological, ecological, and social forces. Believe that one achieves **well-being** by securing a peaceful relationship with the supernatural world.
10. Filipinos (Daisy Rodriguez, Carolina De Guzman, and Arthur Cantos): Illness is caused by **imbalance** of "hot"/"cold" and air elements in body. Filipinos may associate illness with bad behavior or punishment. Prevent illness by avoiding inappropriate behaviors that cause **imbalance**, and cure illness by avoiding inappropriate behaviors that cause **imbalance**, and cure illness by restoring **balance.**

11. Haitians (Jessie Colin): Maintaining **equilibrium** and praying are essential for good health. Achieving a healthy **balance** requires good spiritual habits.

12. Hawaiians (Donna-Marie Palakiko): According to ancient beliefs, the body is a vessel for God and house for spirits. **Disharmony**, loss of power *(mana)*, or loss of **balance** between a person and god, other humans, and the land are causes of illness *(ma'i)*. One regains **balance** through prayer, *ho'oponopono* (setting right, counseling), correcting the cause of the illness, and herbal medicine.

13. Iranians (Homeyra Hafizi): Health is **harmony** of the mind and soul, a state that depends on the interplay and **balance** of factors both within one's control and beyond it.

14. Japanese (Gayle Shiba, Yuko Matsumoto Leong, and Roberta Oka): Naturalistic causes include being out of **balance** from lack of sleep or poor diet. Holistic causes may include loss of spiritual family, or environmental **harmony.**

15. Koreans (Eun-Ok Im): Traditionally, good health is a result of **harmonious** relationships in the human and supernatural worlds, and in the universe at large. The key is maintaining vital energy (ki) and **balance** in all aspects of one's life. **Balancing** yin (um) and yang in diet and other areas of life is particularly important in avoiding illness. Koreans still view health holistically, as a **balanced** state in all aspects of life.

16. Mexicans (Peter Andrew Guarnero): May view physical illness as an act of God—therefore something to be endured—or the result of living a bad life or lifestyle. Persons who are more highly educated tend to perceive physical illness as a sign of an unhealthy lifestyle and within the individual's control. Cultural causes of illness include humoral **imbalance** and folk syndromes such as the evil eye *(mal de ojo)*, fright *(susto)*, and intestinal blockage *(empacho)*.

17. Nigerians (Marcellina Ada Ogbu): View health from a holistic perspective, as a state of **harmony** with one's environment, including the supernatural world (gods, ancestors' spirits, and deities). Disease is the result of **disharmony** and conflict.

18. Pakistanis (Saleema S. Hashwani): Traditional humoral belief holds that "hot"/"cold" **imbalances** cause sickness; hot/cold qualities describe food, drinks, medicinal herbs, individual human nature, and specific illnesses.

19. Puerto Ricans (Tereza C. Juarbe): Hereditary factors, lack of personal attention to health, **humoral imbalance**, or negative environmental forces, such as toxins, cause illness.

20. Samoans (John Mayer, Dianne Ishida, and Tusitala Feagaiga Toomata-Mayer): Samoans believe that illness may be of European origin *(ma'i palagi)* or Samoan origin *(ma'i Samoa)*. **Imbalances** in physical, spiritual, and mental **harmony** requires a holistic approach to healing.

21. Vietnamese (Thu T. Nowak): Many believe that poor health results from yin-yang *(am-duong)* **imbalance**. Some attribute illness to naturalistic causes, such as spoiled food or inclement weather.

22. Yugoslavians (Alma Alikadic): Natural causes include **imbalances** in daily living, such as poor eating habits, cold weather and wind, dirty or contaminated environments, too much stress, trying too hard to make a decent living, and recently, war-related circumstances.

KEY CONCEPTS:

1. Culture is the product of a highly adaptive and superior human brain.
2. Culture is a patterned response that developed over time and became imprinted in various social, religious, and artistic manifestations.
3. Basic characteristics of culture are: 1) Culture is learned and passed from generation to generation, 2) It is social in nature in that it involves interactions among human beings, 3) It is dynamic, adaptive, and ever-changing.
4. Health and illness concepts are elements of balance that are imbedded in cultural beliefs and practices throughout the world. Allopathic and homeopathic models of medical care are two major dominant health philosophies recognized and practiced in modern era.
5. Harmony of mind and body is essential in preserving balance and health. These beliefs are embodied in the opposite but complementary aspects of the yin and yang philosophy in most Asian cultures. The energy "chi" is believed in some Asian cultures as the internal force that creates harmony and balance between the mind and body and maintains a person's overall health.
6. Balance concepts are imbedded in cultural beliefs and practices, not just in health and illness, but also extends to many aspects of life such as activities of daily living, food practices, medicine, childbirth, child-bearing, healing, spiritual beliefs, supernatural beliefs, etc. Balance appears to be a common thread in the cultural fabric of human life.
7. Balance concepts are contained in cultural beliefs of many people around the world, whether these are specifically identified or implied in written literature. Authors from over twenty different cultures throughout the world have identified balance concepts in their health and illness beliefs.

CHAPTER 5: BALANCE AND CULTURE

REFERENCES

1. Wells, S. 2003. *The Journey of Man*. New York. Random House Trade Paperbacks.
2. Daniels, R., Grendell, R.N. and Wilkins, F.R. 2004. *Nursing Fundamentals: Caring and Clinical Decision Making*. New York. Delmar Thomson. p. 90-112.
3. Giger, J.N. and Davidhizar, R.E. 1995. *Transcultural Nursing* (2ⁿᵈ ed.) St. Louis, Missouri. Mosby-Year Book, Inc., p. 3.
4. Leininger, M. 1985. *Qualitative Research Methods in Nursing*. Orlando, Fla. Grune & Stratton.
5. Spector, R. 1991. *Cultural Diversity in Health and Illness* (3ʳᵈ ed.) Norwalk, CT. Appleton & Lange.
6. Boyle, J. and Andrews, M. 1989. *Transcultural Concepts in Nursing Care*. Glenview, Ill. Scott. Foresman.
7. Purnell, L.D. and Paulanka, B.J. 2003. *Transcultural Health Care: A Culturally Competent Approach* (2ⁿᵈ ed.) Philadelphia. F.A. Davis.
8. Spector, R. 2009. *Cultural Diversity in Health and Illness* (7ᵗʰ ed.) Upper Saddle River, NJ. Pearson Prentice Hall.
9. Edlin, G., Golanty,E., and Brown, K.M. 1999. *Health and Wellness* (6ᵗʰ ed.) Sudbury, MA. Jones and Bartlett Publishers, Inc.
10. Lipson, J.G. and Dibble, S.L.(Eds.) 2005. *Culture and Clinical Care*. San Francisco, CA: UCSF School of Nursing Press.

PART II

BALANCE IN HEALTH
AND NURSING

Chapter 6

THE HEALTH-ILLNESS
BALANCE CONTINUUM

"The chief condition on which, life, health, and vigor depends on, is action. It is by action that an organism develops its faculties, increases its energy, and attains the fulfillment of its destiny."
—Colin Powell

An essential element for continued survival is the preservation of good health. As one of the core elements of balance, health is the underlying supporting matrix that enables human beings to sustain itself, thereby making it possible to achieve homeostasis, maintain equilibrium, adapt to changing conditions, and meet its needs within its internal and external environments. Health is not static. It is a dynamic state or condition influenced by many factors both within and outside the human body. The fluidity of this state is not only in the physical body; it is also a state influenced by the mind. A balanced state is a result of the dynamic interaction between two opposite forces—the force of positive energy, and the force of negative energy. Positive forces bring about health and well-being; negative forces bring decreased well-being and illness. Attitudes, beliefs, and mental states affect the way people perceive their state of health and their health behaviors. Seeking balance is key to achieving equilibrium, good health, and ultimately, a meaningful existence and survival. Man is able to fulfill his destiny if enjoying good physical, mental and spiritual health.

The opposite of good health is illness, a state of imbalance brought about by many causes—infection, extreme temperatures, trauma, cancerous growth, toxic chemicals, malnutrition, dehydration, emotional upset, etc. Illness affects not just the physical body but also the mental state of well-being of the individual. Illness reflects the direct relationship between the individual and the internal and external environment. The outside environment is replete with noxious elements that can potentially cause illness, such as carbon dioxide, fire, smoke, toxic gases, contaminated food and water, ultra-violet rays from the sun, etc. Likewise, an imbalance in the internal environment of the body can bring about illness—such as electrolyte disturbances, dehydration, infection, malnutrition, and other disease processes. Inability of the body to neutralize the harmful effects of these elements and processes to bring the body back to its normal state of balance can lead to further deterioration, severe imbalances, and even death. The consequences of physical and mental imbalances are manifested in the degree of illness.

The process of bringing the body back to a state of balance from an illness or imbalance is known as ***healing.*** The body is already endowed by nature to heal itself through regenerative physical properties of the cells and organs of the body. It has the capacity to protect itself through thick outer coverings such as the skin and skull, thereby protecting the internal structures underneath. It has a built-in protective array of cells throughout the body to fight off invading foreign bodies that cause harm. Compensatory mechanisms exist in the body to offset deficits and continue to enable the body to maintain balance and thus survive. Most of all, the human brain is such a complex machine that can adjust its mental processes to deal with physical limitations through balance-seeking behaviors. It appears that the body is built to maintain balance through numerous and redundant processes and capabilities. It can adapt itself to various circumstances. This adaptive and protective capacity is one of the great mysteries of human life that has yet to be fully understood.

DEFINITIONS OF HEALTH

What is **health?** Leading authorities have various definitions of this concept. A foremost definition is one by the World Health Organization that defined health in 1946 as "a state of complete physical, mental and social well-being and not merely the absence of disease or infirmity".[1] Although this definition has been the subject of considerable debate, this definition has remained the most enduring. The difficulty with accepting this definition is that it seems to suggest a static state where health is achieved only when a "complete" state of physical, mental and social well-being is attained. However, it also qualifies this state by adding that it is not merely the absence of disease or infirmity. It seems to suggest that there are other dimensions of health beyond the absence of disease or infirmity.

A Webster dictionary definition of health is "physical and mental well-being, freedom from disease, etc".[2] Again, this appears to be a narrow definition that does not account for the social well-being aspect of health.

Mosby has a broader definition of health that expands the WHO definition as a condition of physical, mental, and social well-being and the absence of disease or other abnormal conditions. It is not a static condition but a constant change and adaptation to stress resulting in homeostasis. Furthermore, it cites Rene Dubos, an author often quoted in nursing education that, "The states of health or disease are the expressions of the success or failure experienced by the organism in its efforts to respond adaptively to environmental challenges". This definition places emphasis on the dynamic quality of health and the essential role of adaptation to health.[3]

The connection between health and balance is central in Spector's definition. A well—respected author on cultural diversity in health and illness, she defines health within the context of balance between the person's internal being and the outside world or external environment. Health is defined as "the balance of a person, both within one's being—physical, mental, and spiritual—and in the outside an imbalance world—natural, familial and communal, and metaphysical."[4] Illness is considered an imbalance of the person both within one's being and with the outside world. Healing is the restoration of balance. She considers the relationship of the person to the outside world as reciprocal.

This definition establishes the larger view of health as an interplay and balancing of factors both within the person's physical and spiritual being and influences in the external environment. The latter includes not just the natural and physical world of material objects but also social factors such as family, community, and society. These are the elements within one's culture that are preserved and passed on through generations. Enduring elements of culture are preserved while others change as relationships, beliefs, attitudes, as well as advances in science and technology change. A decade ago, social networking via the internet was unheard of. Now, people in the modern world, influenced by advanced technology that emanated from the Western world, are interacting with each other differently via the internet. Who would have thought that we would witness such a revolutionary change during our lifetime? Certainly, culture has changed in this modern era. Access to health information is now widely available to people all over the world and it is changing health attitudes, beliefs, and habits.

Daniels, et al view health as a process through which an individual seeks equilibrium, an element of balance, to promote stability and comfort. They acknowledge that it is a dynamic process that varies according to the person's perception of well-being. Illness, on the other hand, is the inability of the individual's adaptive responses to maintain physical and emotional balance. They describe balance as referring to homeostasis, a state of equilibrium among psychological, physiological, sociocultural, intellectual, and spiritual needs. It includes the concept of adaptation, described as the process by which a person adjusts to achieve homeostasis.[5]

This view of health addresses all aspects of the individual person's life that includes the following: physical status, emotional well-being, social relationships, intellectual functioning, and spiritual condition. This is a holistic view that takes into consideration all aspects of the human condition from the individual person's perspective. It considers the external environment as a major factor influencing the person's health and well-being. It is valuable in the sense that it recognizes that seeking equilibrium or balance is a goal of health. The lack of ability of the person to respond adaptively to maintain physical and emotional balance can result in illness. Adaptation to changes appear to be essential in maintaining this balance. This involves behaviors that are balance-seeking in order to achieve an optimum level of health.

Pender, known for her **Health Promotion Model**, along with colleagues Murdaugh and Parsons, define health in terms of individual characteristics, behavior-specific knowledge and affect, and behavioral outcomes.[6] Each person has specific and unique personal characteristics and experiences that affect their behavioral outcomes. These are individual variables that can be modified through interventions or actions by a professional nurse. Health-promoting behavior is the desired outcome of the Health Promotion Model. Potter and Perry [7] appears to concur with this view. For the nurse to help clients identify and reach their health goals, information about the client's life conditions and concepts of health must be determined.

A broader definition by Murray and Zentner is more closely aligned with the balance concept which defines health as "purposeful, adaptive response, physically, mentally, emotionally, and socially, to internal and external stimuli in order to maintain stability and comfort". [8] In this definition, adaptation, one of the core elements of the balance concept, is manifested through adaptive responses (behavior) in response to the internal and external stimuli (environmental elements), to maintain stability (equilibrium) and comfort (well-being).

Components of the Health Definition

From these various views and definitions, a certain pattern appears to emerge: that health has different components that all contribute to a more comprehensive understanding of the health concept. First, that health is a **dynamic process** and not a static one; second, a sense of **well-being** must be present for the individual to be considered healthy; third, that the element of **balance** pervades the process of achieving health. As Daniels suggests, individuals seeks equilibrium, a core element of balance, to achieve stability. Fourth, that health is totally **individual**, that the variables that determine a person's state of health differ from one person to another. This results in behaviors that are unique to the individual according to their perceptions, beliefs, attitudes, physical capacities, and experiences as Pender and colleagues suggest. The human tendency is to seek balance through behaviors that may or may not contribute to health and well-being. Health professionals can assist individuals in performing **health-promoting** behaviors, a manifestation of balance-seeking. Fifth, factors both within the individual and the outside **environment**, predominantly the person's **culture**, influence health status, attitudes, beliefs and behavior. Culture is a major determinant of health as espoused by major authors. Many cultures around the world have engrained balance concepts in their health and spiritual beliefs and practices as discussed in the previous chapter.

It seems that a more comprehensive definition of health is necessary in order to better understand all the dimensions of this concept. A **holistic** approach is perhaps the best way to understand this difficult concept. While each author's definition has its own merit, it is like looking at different reflections of a prism. By taking a broader view of health in terms of the underlying concept of balance and its core elements, health could be better understood more fully. *Balance brings all these various views together through the prism of its core elements: homeostasis, adaptation, equilibrium, needs, and health.* All of these elements are essential for human survival achieved through balance-seeking behaviors. Ultimately, health is one of the core elements of balance that contribute to the optimal well-being and survival of human beings.

A definition of health must include the **mental health** aspect and is stressed in the WHO's definition of health. Mental health is defined as a state of well-being in which every individual realizes his or her own potential, can cope with the normal stresses of life, can work productively and fruitfully, and is able to make a contribution to her or his community.[9] This recognizes that psychological stress plays a major role in the mental health and well-being of individuals. How each person deals with and manages stress depends on many variables that differ from one person to another. This determines the coping strategies the person uses. Two kinds of stress were identified by Selye:[10] *distress,* or harmful stress, and *eustress*, stress that is conducive to health. In this context, many of the stresses of modern life are harmful and could be termed distress. The daily grind of every day modern life can produce harmful stresses that affect mental well-being. These include work stress, family stress, relationship stress, environmental stress, and unfulfilled role expectations within the society of which a person is part. Cultural standards and expectations can produce stress on members of the group especially if one deviates from the accepted norms. Eustress, such as brought about by religion and spiritual beliefs can provide psychological and mental respite for a person's stress. Positive experiences that produce physiological and psychological stress responses can be beneficial to the body, such as the stress of physical exercise.

HEALTH, WELLNESS AND ILLNESS: A CONTINUUM

Health, wellness, and illness are concepts that are generally viewed as a continuum, defined as "a continuous whole".[11] Health and illness are opposite states, in the same way as the concepts of balance and imbalance. They are concepts that are opposite each other, quite distinct in their own properties and yet, one cannot be conceived or understood without the other. This polarity of opposites is the underlying concept in the Chinese philosophy of "yin and yang". Many dualities that exist in nature are thought to be manifestations of the yin and yang. Paradoxically, opposites in this philosophy have to coexist and viewed as a whole. One cannot be understood without understanding the other. Much of the human existence is dominated by this philosophy. Without the existence of one state, the opposite condition cannot be appreciated. Within the continuum, there are varying degrees of either one of these states, such as different degrees of wellness defined by the individual.

Wellness is a concept that is closely intertwined with the health and illness concepts. Wellness describes the health status not just qualitatively but also quantitatively. *Wellness is a feeling state of optimal level of health as experienced and lived by the individual.* If health is a state of balance or equilibrium and illness is a state of imbalance, wellness is the state that starts at the optimal level of health and is absent in extreme illness. Wellness acts as the supporting beam that runs along the continuum from optimal health to critical illness. The essence of wellness is balance.

The health-wellness-illness continuum is illustrated in this diagram based on Daniel's "Health continuum" diagram.[12]

THE HEALTH-WELLNESS-ILLNESS CONTINUUM

<u>DEGREES OF BALANCE :</u>

BALANCE---IMBALANCE

Zone of equilibrium

<u>DEGREES OF WELLNESS/ILLNESS</u>:

Optimal health—Good health—Normal health—Mild illness/Poor health—Critical illness/Death

The opposite of health is illness; the opposite of balance is imbalance. However, it is easier to measure illness than it is to measure health. Illness can be measured using parameters and quantitative measures, such as laboratory tests, as an indication of illness or lack of it. Abnormal findings or results determine the degree or acuteness of the illness. But how do you measure health? Health assessments reveal data about the individual that are both subjective and objective. One example is pain. How do you measure pain? The primary measure of pain is the individual's description of the degree or intensity of it. Subjective data are the individual's self-report of the symptom. And subjective symptoms are based on the individual's perceptions, feelings, emotions, experiences, attitudes, personality make-up, developmental stage, cultural background, socio-economic status, health beliefs and attitudes, spirituality, etc. Communication patterns contribute to the description of the subjective symptoms and these vary from individual to individual. Herein lies the difficulty at arriving at a common definition that applies to everybody.

Normal health is the goal of human existence. It is that state where balance and equilibrium is lived, felt, and strived for by human beings in all aspects of their existence—physical, mental, spiritual, and psychosocial. Wellness is a dynamic process which constantly changes, whether the individual is consciously aware of it or not. A well person may have a certain degree of illness; an ill person may have certain degree of wellness. A person may feel "well" physically but may not be well emotionally. Physical illness affects a person's emotional state; emotional illness affects the person's physical being. The mind-body influences on each other are always at work to help maintain this balance state. Normal coping mechanisms or adaptive responses enable individuals to deal with factors that affect their health and achieve a state of normalcy or equilibrium. When individuals are no longer able to utilize those physical and psychological mechanisms to achieve balance, then a state of imbalance or illness occurs.

Health is also understood in the context of balance maintenance, promotion, and restoration. The view of health as a process through which an individual seeks equilibrium that promotes stability and comfort is frequently found in literatures. That health is a dynamic process is also well-accepted, which generally includes balance of all human aspects: physical, psychological, socio-cultural, intellectual, and spiritual. This state of equilibrium includes balance both with the internal and external environments. Some equate equilibrium with **homeostasis**, although this term usually refers to the relative constancy in the internal environment maintained by adaptive physiologic responses that promote healthy survival. The process that the body adjusts to the changes within his/her body and to the changes in the external environment directly affecting it is called ***adaptation.*** All these elements of balance work together to preserve life and health of the human being. How do these processes translate to an identifiable and measurable state of health? The answer may be in the link between beliefs and attitudes and behaviors. However, knowing the myriad of factors that intervene between mental process and behavior, it is not difficult to understand this dilemma. Models of health help to clarify these relationships.

MODELS OF HEALTH AND ILLNESS

In order to better understand the concepts of health and illness, models have been developed by various authors. Models are theoretical ways of understanding a concept or idea and help to understand their meanings in relation to other concepts. Models of health and illness are used to understand these concepts in relation to health attitudes, behaviors and outcomes. There are several theoretical models of health which are all intended to clarify the relationship between health, wellness, illness, and human behavior. The following are several models of health and their highlights:

The **Health belief model** (HBM)[13] is a psychological model that attempts to explain and predict health behaviors. This is done by focusing on the attitudes and beliefs of individuals. The HBM was first developed in the 1950s by social psychologists Hochbaum, Rosenstock and Kegels working in the U.S. Public Health Services. The model is based on the assumptions that expectations direct human behaviors that lead to the fulfillment of these expectations and that health beliefs, which may change as the person develops, are influenced by group values.

High level wellness model (Dunn)[14] is oriented toward maximizing the highest health potential of an individual. In order to achieve one's full potential, the individual must maintain a continuum of balance and purposeful direction within the environment.

Health Promotion Model (Pender)[15] known as HPM. This model proposed by Nola Pender in 1982 and revised in 1996 synthesizes research findings from nursing, psychology and public health. It describes the multifaceted nature of human beings as they interact within their environment to pursue health. This model focuses on three basic components: 1) unique characteristics and experiences of each person, 2) behavior-specific knowledge and affect, 3) behavioral outcomes. The third one is achieved through health-promoting behaviors that results in good health. Nursing actions can help individuals modify behavior to achieve positive outcomes.

Basic Human Needs Model is based on Abraham Maslow's Hierarchy of Needs. The concept of human needs in this model has been used in nursing as basis for applying nursing care and was discussed in the first chapter of this book. According to this model, needs are arranged in a hierarchical fashion with the basic physiological needs first, followed by higher level psychosocial needs such as safety and security, love and belonging, self-esteem, and self-actualization as the highest level of need. Basic human needs are those that are necessary for human health and physical survival. Needs have to be met according to what is most operational at a given moment. Higher needs take precedence once lower needs are met.

Holistic Health Models are those models that consider all dimensions of the person—physical, emotional, mental, psychosocial, and spiritual—to achieve the highest form of well-being and optimal health. This view of health has gained more acceptance over the years as the importance of a more integrated approach to caring for clients began to be recognized. This approach is more client-centered and takes into consideration the unique dimensions of each individual.

THE HEALTH-ILLNESS BALANCE CONTINUUM

An alternative view of health as a dynamic state along the axis of balance and imbalance in the health-illness continuum is a core concept in this book. It is presented in the *"HEALTH-ILLNESS BALANCE CONTINUUM"* as a conceptual model of health, illness, and balance (Diagram 6.1). This model is based on the following assumptions:

1. Health and illness are opposing states of the human being that exist in a continuum that are dynamic and may change from a state of balance (optimal health) to a state of imbalance (illness), or vice versa.
2. Health is a state maintained by the body as a natural tendency to achieve stability and equilibrium within the internal and external environment. This state can fluctuate from minimal health, moderate health, and optimal health. Optimal health is achieved within the **"Zone of Equilibrium"**, a state of complete balance, well-being, stability, and normalcy.
3. A person's state of health always moves along a **vertical axis of balance and imbalance** with optimal health within the balance zone of equilibrium at the top, and disease states or imbalance towards the bottom on the opposite end. That state is subject to change at any time and as defined by the individual. One's state of health becomes more balanced as one moves upward along the axis towards the zone of equilibrium. Moving away from the zone of equilibrium means moving towards imbalance and a state of illness.
3. Health and Illness are on opposite ends of the balance-imbalance axis. Health is a state of balance and ranges from minimum health, moderate health and optimal health. Illness is a state of imbalance and ranges from mild to moderate to severe states, leading to death if irreversible.
4. An individual's behaviors, lifestyle, inherited characteristics, and environment determine factors that have positive or negative effects on their state of health. Positive factors are balance-producing; negative factors are imbalance-producing. A balanced lifestyle contributes to optimal health.
5. Behaviors that are balance-seeking contribute to optimal health; balance-negating behaviors contribute to illness.

6. Medical and nursing interventions can reverse a state of illness or imbalance to a state of health or balance through behavioral and attitude modifications and treatments.

This author is of the view that an individual's "state of health" is a dynamic interplay of numerous factors within his internal environment and the world outside his body. This state of health is not static. The body needs to constantly monitor internal conditions and receive information from the outside environment in order for the body to stay within the **"Zone of Equilibrium"**, a state of optimal balance and health. Within this zone of balance or optimal health, all the internal and external forces are in complete balance with each other at a given point in time; all the indicators of bodily functions are within normal range. In this model, the view of the health and illness as a continuum is consistent with existing models, with wellness and health on one end of the continuum and illness and death on the opposite end. However, instead of a parallel line, this continuum runs from top to bottom with **optimal health, the highest level of health at the top, and states of illness at the opposite bottom**. *This concept of the health-illness continuum runs along an imaginary **vertical axis** of balance and imbalance from top to bottom, instead of a parallel line across. **This is what is unique about this model.*** This puts the highest level of health at the top most, which is the goal of balance-seeking. The opposite end of this axis is imbalance, or states of illness which can range from mild to severe. Irreversible imbalances lead to death. One's state of health or balance is dynamic and can change anytime, which also changes its location along the axis.

Because the state of health is in a constant state of flux, this balance could be changed by any negative force impinging on the individual. The individual can move from the zone of equilibrium along the axis continuum down to a state of imbalance at any given time. A sudden accident or major trauma can completely throw a healthy person into a state of imbalance; any major life event such as sudden death in the family may put a normally coping person into depression, a state of mental imbalance. Acute, persistent or chronic imbalance can cause illness or disease. Uncontrolled environmental factors such extreme weather conditions, disasters, fire, tsunamis, exposure to dangerous chemicals, or infectious diseases can cause illnesses and even death.

Levels of health are in a continuum as do levels of illness. People define health as a state of being according to their own values, personality and lifestyle. Many factors influence a person's health and/or illness behaviors. These factors could be either positive or negative in relation to their effects on producing, maintaining or restoring a balanced lifestyle. Individual variables mediate a person's health behaviors and these originate from two sources: 1) innate or occurring naturally, such as inherited traits, personality, and developmental stage, and 2) acquired, or obtained externally, such as environment, culture and society.

The degree of these illness conditions can range from mild to moderate to extreme. Similarly, health and wellness can range from minimal health, to moderate health, to optimum health—the highest level of wellness. This is where a complete state of balance and equilibrium exists. Minimal health is when the body is barely able to maintain its functions but do not outwardly demonstrate any imbalances. The line between minimal health and illness may not be well-defined. In a moderate state of health, all indicators are within normal range. For all intents and purposes, this is a healthy individual but it takes more energy to maintain a state of wellness. An optimal state of health is when the individual performs at his/her highest capacity and uses all available resources to maximize his/her potentials to achieve a perfect balance in life. This is comparable to Maslow's self-actualization level.

To maintain a state of health from minimal to optimal requires a certain balance between the positive and negative forces that are always impinging on the individual. Positive forces are those factors that contribute to health and wellness: healthy behaviors, good diet, exercise, mental and emotional stability, etc. Negative forces are those factors that contribute to imbalances, such as risky behaviors, disease, trauma, and stresses (physical, psychological and sociological). A balanced lifestyle consists of those behaviors that augment positive factors and diminish negative factors.

Because of the dynamic interplay of positive and negative forces within the human system, negative forces can negate the effects of balance and result in an imbalance, or a state of illness. Mild and moderate illness states can be more easily reversed through medical and nursing interventions and adopting healthier lifestyles and behaviors. Severe states of illness may get to the point of irreversibility and lead to death, regardless of any intervention. Health-seeking behaviors and attitudes are positive forces that help the individual to return to a state of health that could be as close to optimal health as possible. *Health-seeking behaviors within the realms of the Behavior Pyramid ultimately enable the individual to achieve the highest physical and psychosocial level: the Self—fulfillment level. This is where one finds the ultimate of balance: the Zone of Equilibrium within the health-illness continuum.*

ROLE OF HEALTH CARE PROFESSIONALS

The role of healthcare professionals in reversing imbalances and return individuals back to a state of balance and equilibrium is crucial in the balance—health equation. The Health-Illness Balance Continuum model establishes the direct link between balance and health. This model provides a conceptual framework in understanding health-seeking behaviors. The formula is simple: by recognizing positive and negative behaviors that either contribute to, or negate balance, health care providers can design individualized interventions that will promote health, well-being and balance. The role of health-seeking behaviors in achieving, maintaining, and restoring health is central to this model. There are many different health professionals who play various roles in the care of patients. Regardless of the setting—hospitals, homes, or community-based—health professionals like nurses, physicians, physical therapists, dieticians, social workers, etc. all contribute to the health and well-being of patients. The Health-Illness Balance continuum provides a common framework towards a greater understanding of the range of health and illness behaviors contributing to balanced or imbalanced states of health. Behaviors that contribute to imbalances can be changed or managed; behaviors that contribute to balance can be reinforced. It takes into consideration factors that are universal to human behavior such as culture, environments, society, nature, inherited characteristics, personality, technology, etc. Ultimately, this helps establish a common platform of understanding of health by health care professionals applicable to every individual living on the planet.

KEY CONCEPTS

1. Health is one of the core elements of the concept of balance that is necessary for survival. It is a dynamic state influenced by many factors both within the internal and external environment of the body. Optimal health is a state of balance brought about by the dynamic interaction of positive and negative forces. Positive forces bring health and well-being; negative forces bring illness and decreased well-being.
2. Illness is a state of imbalance, the opposite of optimal health. As in health, illness is also influenced by factors both within the internal and the external environment. The degree of illness is a reflection of the body's inability to correct imbalances and neutralize the harmful effects of those elements that cause the imbalance.
3. The process of healing can bring the body back from a state of imbalance to a state of balance through innate regenerative, corrective, and protective mechanisms of the body. Balance-seeking behaviors enable the human being to seek balance through actions that promote health and well-being.
4. Health has been defined in different ways by various authorities, and the World Health Organization. Other definitions consider culture as a major component of health; others focus on balance and equilibrium. Still others consider behavior, adaptive responses, and environment as part of their health definition. All these elements are considered part of a comprehensive and holistic view of health. Mental health and the role of stress in mental health are important aspects of the health concept.
5. Health, illness, and wellness are viewed as a continuum consistent with the balance-imbalance concepts. This view exists in the Asian philosophy of the duality of the "yin" and "yang". Manifestations of this duality are evident in many aspects of human life. Many cultural beliefs and practices have their roots in this duality philosophy. Wellness is the state of optimal health. Degrees of wellness range from optimal health to critical illness and death. The essence of wellness is balance.

6. Models have been developed in order to better understand the concepts of health, wellness, and illness in relation to other concepts such as health promotion, health beliefs, human needs, and other human dimensions. Examples are the Health Belief Model (HBM), Health promotion Model (HPM), Basic Human Needs Model, and Holistic Health Model.

7. The key concepts of the Health-Illness Balance Continuum model are the following: 1) Health and illness are dynamic opposing states that exist in a continuum and constantly change to maintain stability within a "zone of equilibrium", a state of optimum balance, well-being, normalcy, and stability, 2) Individual factors influenced by the external environment determine individual behaviors that have positive or negative effects on their state of health, 3) Balance-seeking behaviors contribute to optimal health while balance-negating behaviors contribute to illness, 4) Medical and nursing interventions can reverse illness or a state of imbalance through behavioral and attitude modifications.

8. The Health-illness Balance Continuum Model is unique in that it views balance and imbalance as health and illness states in a continuum along a **vertical axis**. The state of health or balance of an individual is dynamic and can change anytime, which also changes its location along the axis.

9. This view of the dynamic relationship between health, illness and balance can serve as the common framework for health professionals in providing individualized care for people of all cultures around the world.

CHAPTER 6: THE HEALTH-ILLNESS BALANCE CONTINUUM

REFERENCES

1. World Health Organization (1946). *Preamble to the constitution of the World Health Organization* as adopted by the International Health Conference, New York, 19-22 June, 1946; signed on 22 July 1946 by the representatives of 61 States (Official Records of the World Health Organization, no. 2, p. 100) and entered into force on 7 April 1948.

2. Agnes, M. (Ed.) and Laird, C. 2002.*Webster's New Dictionary and Thesaurus.* Cleveland, Ohio. Wiley Publishing, Inc., p.293.

3. Mosby Elsevier. 2006. *Mosby's Dictionary of Medicine, Nursing & Health Professions* (7th ed.) St. Louis, Missouri. Mosby, Inc., p.853

4. Spector, R.E. 2009. *Cultural Diversity in Health and Illness* (7th ed.) Upper Saddle River, New Jersey. Pearson Prentice Hall.

5. Daniels, R., et al. 2010. *Nursing Fundamentals: Caring and Clinical Decision Making* (2nd ed.) Clifton Park, NY. Delmar, p. 962-964.

6. Pender, N.J., Murdaugh, C.L. & Parsons, M.A. 2002. *Health Promotion in Nursing Practice* (4th ed.). Upper Saddle River, NJ. Prentice Hall.

7. Potter, P.A. and Perry, A.G. 2005. *Fundamentals of Nursing* (6th ed.) St. Louis, Missouri. Mosby.

8. Murray, R. and Zentner, J. 1975. *Nursing Concepts for Health Promotion.* Englewood Cliffs, NJ. Prentice Hall.

9. World Health Organization. *Mental Health: a State of Well-being.* http://www.who.int/features/factfiles/mental_health/en/index.html.(retrieved 3/24/2012).

10. Potter, P.A. and Perry, A.G. 2007. *Basic Nursing: Essentials for Practice* (6th ed.) St. Louis, Missouri. Mosby.

11. Agnes, M. (Ed.) and Laird, C. 2002.*Webster's New Dictionary and Thesaurus.* Cleveland, Ohio. Wiley Publishing, Inc., p.135.

12. Daniels, R., et al. 2010. *Nursing Fundamentals: Caring and Clinical Decision Making* (2nd ed.) Clifton Park, NY. Delmar, p.965.

13. Health Belief Model. http://www.utwente.nl/cw/theorieenoverzicht/theoryclusters/healthco. (retrieved 1/10/2013).

14. RNpedia—*Health and illness.* http://www.rnpedia.com/home/notes/fundamentals-of-nursing-notes/health. (retrieved 1/9/2013).

15. Nola J. Pender—*Health Promotion Model*. Cardinal Stritch University Library. http://www. library.stritch.edu/research/subjects/health/nursingTheorists/pender. (retrieved 3/24/2012.

DIAGRAM 6.1 THE HEALTH ILLNESS BALANCE CONTINUUM

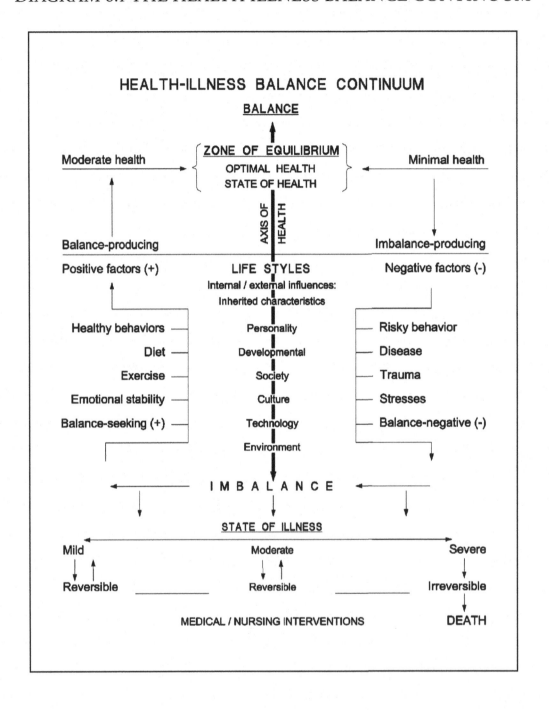

Chapter 7

THEORETICAL UNDERPINNINGS IN NURSING

"Even if there is only one possible unified theory, it is just a set of rules and equations. What is it that breathes fire into the equations and makes a universe for them to describe?
—Stephen Hawking*

The concepts of balance and its core elements are found in nursing literatures and are essential components in nursing theories. The concepts of balance, imbalance, homeostasis, health, equilibrium, adaptation, behavior, environment, culture, and open systems are all within the global view of nursing and healthcare. Nursing's view of its profession is holistic, in that it considers, not just disease processes and its treatments, but also the factors that contribute to the health and illness of their clients. These factors are within all human dimensions: its physical self and its internal mechanisms of structure and function; the mind and how it affects behavior; the development of personality and age-dependent behaviors; the influence of the internal environment and external environment on health and human behavior in an open system; physiologic and psychosocial needs; the spiritual aspect; the influence of culture on beliefs, attitude and behavior; and the influence of society on man as a social being.

It becomes obvious that behavior plays a central part in defining the human being. Behavior enables human beings to respond to innate internal stimuli, as well as manipulate the external environment to achieve stability and survival. The energy or impetus that propels humans to act in certain ways is dictated by a need to achieve balance and equilibrium, and eventually, preserve itself from extinction. Without the energy of balance, survival will not be possible. Behavior is the key that unlocks the potential energy of the five pillars of balance: homeostasis, adaptation, equilibrium, needs and health.

Modern nursing has evolved from its early beginnings when Florence Nightingale planted the seeds of a new way of caring for people. Nursing is a caring profession that is centered around the care of clients. The health and welfare of the client are its reasons for being. To Nightingale, caring for clients include attention to the external physical environment, because it affects client's health and well-being. In her "Notes on Nursing",[1] she emphasized the importance of environmental sanitation, clean air, good ventilation, keeping the clients warm and comfortable, good hygiene, cleanliness, pure water, among other things. Her philosophy of nursing is based on health maintenance and restoration—still the pillars of nursing care today. She believed in the effects of the mind on the body—the foundations of mental health. While she did not specifically mention the concept of balance, the rudiments of balance are in her writings—like maintaining appropriate body temperature, the benefits of sunlight as opposed to darkness in healing, cold air as opposed to warm air, the harmful effects of environment such as smoke and foul smell, the need for food and good nutrition, the importance of keeping mental harmony and stability to healing. Fundamentally, she was client-centered and believed in nursing interventions for the healing and restoration of the client's health.

EVOLUTION OF NURSING AND MEDICINE

It is important to study the history of nursing as it developed along with the medical profession because it places in perspective the close relationship between the two professions. Health and illness are the basic foundations common to medicine and nursing. The two professions are closely linked together, not just historically, but also in the philosophies they share about health and illness. In, fact, the "Florence Nightingale Pledge"[2] often used by nurses during graduation ceremonies, is an adaptation of the Hippocratic Oath taken by physicians. The evolution of nursing and medicine actually started early in the history of human civilization. However, medicine as a profession outpaced the development of nursing. Nursing as a science is a relatively young field compared to medicine. The practice of medicine can be found in the ancient histories of Egypt, Greece, Babylonia, India and China.[3] The use of plants for medicinal purposes dates back to the prehistoric ages. It is said that the Egyptians and Babylonians both introduced the concepts of diagnosis, prognosis and medical examination—all still in use as standard medical practice today. The Hippocratic Oath, dating back from the 5th century BCE and was written in Greece, is still taken by physicians around the world. As technology and knowledge about health and diseases expanded, medical practice also continued to advance its profession throughout history, focusing on various techniques of treatments, and curing of diseases.

Just as medicine evolved from its ancient beginnings, so did nursing. Evidence that nursing was practiced can be traced back to primitive societies as early as 4000 BC.[4] The use of wet nurses was recorded in 2000 BC in Babylonia and Assyria. Nursing caregivers were used in hospitals during the Byzantine era. During the Middle Ages, care of sick people was mostly provided by men who belonged to various religious orders of knights. But it was in India where the strong religious influence on nursing originated between 800 BC and 600 BC.

Societal changes during the Renaissance shifted care from institutions to homes where care of the sick was mostly provided by women who continued their role as nurturers and care-givers. The Industrial Revolution was a dark period in the history of nursing. While medical schools were established in Europe, there were no similar training for nurses. Women who worked in hospitals were mostly alcoholics and prostitutes who were serving jail time. This also served as an impetus later on for nurse reformers like Florence Nightingale to change the negative public image of nursing to a more respectable one. It had to break away from the public perception, some of which may still exist today, that nurses are "handmaidens" to the physician. This process will take over two centuries when nursing eventually evolved into a discipline with a body of scientific knowledge all its own.

DEVELOPMENT OF NURSING THEORIES

A profession's body of knowledge guides its practice.[5] And this body of knowledge is based on sound scientific principles backed by research. It utilizes evidence to support rationale for the practice of the profession. Theories contribute to the development of a substantive body of knowledge required for the practice of a profession. This has been the challenge that the nursing profession has faced since the time that Florence Nightingale began the journey towards professionalism. It is the realization that a knowledge base is required for professional nursing practice, as different from medical practice, which served as strong impetus for the rapid development of nursing theories over the last century. The push for more evidence-based practice utilizing research findings and verifiable data to improve practice outcomes and ensure safety propelled nursing into a science-based discipline.

Existing nursing theories developed over a span of several decades by leading nursing theorists were formulated to achieve differing purposes. Theories may be broad or limited to an area in a discipline that it addresses. These may be: to define or predict relationships between concepts, explain health behaviors, identify variables or factors affecting clients in a health care environment, describe phenomena, provide an overall framework for the practice of nursing, or identify specific interventions. These theories all contribute to the body of knowledge used in today's modern nursing practice. Because nursing practice has a holistic approach, it borrows from other disciplines and fields of study such as medicine, psychology, sociology, physics, chemistry, mathematics, to name some of the major ones. The need for cultural competency in nursing practice has also opened up a whole new way of thinking and approaches. Culture, with its multidimensional aspects, further expanded the discipline of nursing and took it to another level.

Theories are the most concrete component of a discipline formulated to propose actions that guide practice. They fall under essentially two categories related to their scope and are applicable to other disciplines as well: grand theories and middle-range theories.[4] A ***grand theory*** is composed of concepts that are broadest in scope and addresses a wide variety of problems identified within the discipline. It is highly abstract and they propose something that is true or testable. A ***middle-range theory*** has a narrower focus and addresses more concrete phenomena than grand theory. There are other terminologies related to knowledge development in general which are also applied to nursing. These include metaparadigm, paradigm, concepts, conceptual framework, and conceptual models, among other terms.[6] A ***metaparadigm*** is the most abstract form of knowledge in a discipline. It identifies the specific phenomena related to that discipline and provides the main structure to the domain of the discipline. The domain of nursing encompasses the *person, environment, health, and nursing*. A ***paradigm*** is a particular viewpoint or way of thinking within a discipline. It represents a main viewpoint supported by research that addresses various areas of interest within the discipline. The building blocks of theories are ***concepts***, which are mental formulations or ideas of a phenomenon. A group of related concepts form a theory. A ***conceptual framework*** is a mental structure that links concepts together. It is a group of concepts that are broadly defined and organized in a systematic fashion to provide a focus or rationale, and a tool for the integration and interpretation of information.[7] On the other hand, a ***conceptual model*** is a symbolic representation of relationships between concepts in a more concrete way such as diagrams, words, mathematical symbols, or physical material.

BALANCE CONCEPTS IN SELECTED NURSING THEORIES

As the building blocks of nursing theory, concepts serve to identify ideas in a phenomenon and reinforce the particular paradigm or viewpoint within the discipline. These concepts were either independently formulated by nursing theorists, or built upon concepts borrowed from other disciplines. For instance, the Adaptation Model developed by Sister Callista Roy combined the general systems theory with adaptation theory. Roy was earlier influenced by her teacher and mentor, Dorothy Johnson, who developed the **Behavioral Systems Model Systems** theory that also originated from the works of other scientists. In looking at various nursing theories, the balance concept and its different elements are contained or implied in their theoretical formulations. It suggests that elements of the balance concept are found in many nursing theories and have broad application within the discipline of nursing.

Because nursing deals with the health care of human beings—individuals, their families, and communities—it is necessary to look for these elements in the professional practice of nursing. These elements are found in several nursing theories but differ according to their focus. Selected theories are each going to be discussed briefly:[4,5,6] (The related concepts and elements of balance contained in each model are bolded)

Florence Nightingale: Environment Theory

Considered the founder of modern nursing, Florence Nightingale revolutionized the direction and status of the nursing profession. She was born to English aristocratic parents on May 12, 1820 in Florence, Italy, while her parents were on a European tour. As a young woman, she realized her "calling" to be a nurse and was accepted for training at Kaiserworth, Germany, a Protestant religious community with a hospital facility. In 1854 during the Crimean War, she brought trained nurses to Scutari, Turkey to take care of wounded soldiers. It was there where she saw the effects of deplorable environmental conditions that threatened the survival of the sick soldiers. She also realized the importance of formally training and educating nurses. When she went back to London, she then established a teaching institution for nurses at St. Thomas Hospital and King's College Hospital. She was a prodigious writer, spending enormous amount of time writing thousands of letters to friends, acquaintances and influential people championing her causes for societal change. Her most notable work is in her book "Notes on Nursing"[2] where she documented her many interests and observations regarding the effects of environment on patient's health, her philosophy of health, the role of the nurse, nursing education, as well as her views on social change.

Florence Nightingale's major contributions to theory development are her views on health, disease, and the environment. Her theory focused on the **environment**. She considered pure air, pure water, efficient drainage, cleanliness, and light as essential elements of environmental health. Ventilation was particularly important in her theory. Although it may seem that her concept of the environment was mainly physical, it also included those elements that affect emotional/mental health. Aspects of the nurses' role in mental health can be gleaned from her theory. She considered it the nurse's responsibility to protect the patient from upsetting news, limiting visitors, controlling noise, and ensuring adequate sleep.

Nightingale recognized the deleterious effects of environment on health. Although the concept of balance was not specifically mentioned in her writings, her environmental theory includes manipulation of the external environment to maintain good ventilation and warmth to keep the patient's temperature stable. Without using the exact terminology, she was actually referring to health-seeking behaviors that are manifestations of both internal and external balance. Good diet and nutrition, basic elements of survival, were recognized as essential to patient's health and recovery. Assessing and meeting the patient's nutritional needs were tasks she believed were nurses' responsibility.

Her views on **health** and **illness** still have much relevance today. Environmental conditions affect health and this is a concept that is true today as it was during her time. Although she did not believe in the germ theory (which was relatively new at that time), she defined health as being well and using every power that person has to achieve an optimal state. She considered disease as a reparative process that nature instituted. She believed in maintenance of health and prevention of disease through environmental controls and nursing practices. Her insistence on environmental and personal cleanliness, such as daily baths by patients and nurses, and the appropriate handling of human wastes, are important components of her theory. These are now essential practices in the modern healthcare world to prevent the spread of diseases. Nightingale's theory still finds wide application and relevance in many of today's nursing practice.

Betty Neuman: Systems Model (1995)

The Neuman Systems Model is based on general system theory which was originally proposed in the 1940's by biologist Ludwig von Bertalanffy.[8] This theory proposed that elements in a complex organization are open to, and interact with their **environments**. By so doing, they produce results that are greater than the sum of the individual parts. The systems concepts include system-environment boundary, input, output, process, state, hierarchy, goal-directedness, and information. These are the same concepts and principles of organization that underlie various other disciplines such as physics, biology, technology, sociology, etc.

The **Gestalt Theory** provided much of the foundation of this model. Gestalt psychology is a school of thought that originated in Germany which proposes that a psychological phenomenon is perceived as a total configuration or pattern, arising from the relationships among its constituent parts.[7] Behavior is seen as an integrated response to a unitary situation rather than discrete isolated behavioral manifestations. The major concepts of this model includes the following: wholistic client approach, open system, structure, environment, created environment, stressors, lines of defense and resistance, degree of reaction, prevention as intervention and reconstitution.[9] In this model, the core structure consists of basic **survival factors** common to the human species. The client is capable of both **input** and **output** related to **environmental** influences and interacting with the environment by adjusting to it. Functional **harmony or balance** preserves the integrity of the system. **Stressors** are tension-producing stimuli that occur within the boundaries of the human system. An adequate level of health is maintained if the human system is able to successfully cope with stress. Wellness is when the parts of the system interact with **harmony**. Illness is a disharmony which results if certain **needs** are not met. Created environment is the person's unconscious mobilization of all system variables toward system integration, stability, and integrity.[7]

Neuman believes that nursing is a unique profession concerned with the totality or wholeness of the client and all the variables affecting a person's response to **stress.** In Neuman's view, the nurse's perception influences the care given so that the care provider's perceptual field must be assessed to help provide appropriate interventions. **Environment** and **person** are core phenomena of the Neuman Systems Model. Environment is defined as all those internal and external factors that surround and influence the person. The nurse's interventions are those purposeful actions defined by Neuman to help retain, attain, and maintain system stability. There are three levels of prevention: primary, secondary and tertiary. The concept of **adaptation** is also an important element of the model. It is called reconstitution which is a state of adaptation to stimuli that produces stress in the internal and external environment. The Neuman theory defines a total-person model for nursing, incorporating a holistic concept and an **open systems** approach. This model provided an organizing framework that brought together the concepts of the whole person, environment, health, and nursing based on solid theoretical foundations from other disciplines.

Dorothy Johnson: Behavioral System Model (1968)

The basic structure of the Behavioral system Model is patterned after a systems model. Johnson conceptualizes the person as a behavioral system in which the outcome is **behavior** that can be observed. She derived her model from works of various behavioral scientists in psychology, sociology and ethnology. The idea that behaviors are specific patterns in response to stresses from biological, psychological, and sociological sources, are derived from works of various other authors The major concepts of this model include behavior, system and behavioral system, subsystems, **equilibrium** and stressors. There are seven subsystems identified in her model: attachment/ affiliative, dependency, ingestive, eliminative, sexual, achievement, and aggressive/ protective.

According to Johnson, behavioral systems are patterned, repetitive, and purposeful ways of behaving. The person as a behavioral system seeks **stability** and **balance** through adjustments and **adaptations** between the person and his or her **environment.** The concept of **equilibrium** is also an integral part of this model and views it as a state in which the individual is in **harmony** with himself and his environment. It suggests a **balance** of the biological and psychological forces influenced by social forces. Subsystems are parts of the behavioral systems that have activities of their own which are interrelated.

This model views the concept of tension, stressors and equilibrium as related to each other. Tension is defined as a state of disturbance of **equilibrium** that stems from inability or inefficient use of energy, thereby hindering the adaptive process. Tension is a manifestation of disturbance in equilibrium. **Stressors** are internal or external stimuli that produce tension. Stressors or stimuli may be positive or negative. Johnson views nursing as a force external to the client or person acting to preserve the organization of the client's behavior while the client is under stress. It provides mechanisms and resources before and during system balance disturbance (illness). A person is viewed as a behavioral system which can be threatened by strong forces that disturb its **balance** and integrity.

Sister Callista Roy: Adaptation Model (1976)

Roy is a contemporary theorist who first published the Roy Adaptation Model in 1976 and continued to further refine and develop her theory.[10] Assumptions of the Adaptation Model are based on systems theory and human adaptive systems combined. The purposes of **adaptation** are survival, growth, reproduction and mastery. She defines the person as an **adaptive system** in constant interaction with a changing internal and external **environment.** It is a bio—psychosocial being responding to **stimuli** in the environment, which she defines as all conditions and influences that affect the development and behaviors of the person. These environmental stimuli can be classified as *focal, contextual,* or *residual.* Focal stimuli are internal or external factors that most immediately confront the person. Contextual stimuli are all those other stimuli that contribute to the effect of the focal stimuli and not immediately confronting the person, but also need to be addressed. Residual stimuli are environmental factors within or outside the human system but have unclear or non-definitive effects.

According to the Roy Adaptation Model, adaptation is achieved through **coping mechanisms** that may be genetically determined. These are automatic processes acquired through experiences and learning. [11] Coping mechanisms are on two basic levels or **subsystems**: *regulator subsystem* and *cognator subsystem.* The regulator subsystem involves the physiologic systems—neural, chemical and endocrine. The cognator subsystem involves the cognitive-emotional systems: perceptual, information processing, learning, judgment, and emotions. The cognator and regulator subsystems cannot be observed directly. Rather, these are recognized through responses, further categorized into four adaptive modes: *physiological, self-concept, role function*, and *interdependence.* The physiological or physical mode enables the person to respond on the physiologic level to their environment. The self-concept mode enables the person to respond on the psychological and spiritual level. Self-concept consists of the person's physical self and self-image, the personal self which includes the moral-ethical-spiritual self, and the group identity mode. The last mode consists of interpersonal relationships, social milieu and culture.

Role function focuses on the roles that the person plays in society, further subcategorized into three roles: primary, secondary, and tertiary roles carried out through behaviors, either through physical performance, or expressive behaviors, such as feelings and attitudes. Primary role determines the main behaviors of the person during a particular time in life. Secondary roles are those that the person plays to complete tasks associated with a developmental stage and primary role. Tertiary roles, which are generally temporary in nature, are roles related to secondary roles and considered choices that are optional in nature.

The interdependence mode is concerned with relationships with others and emphasizes feelings towards others as well as accepting nurturing, love, respect, and value from other people considered important by the person.

Roy's definition of **health** is closely associated with her adaptation concept, the purposes of which are survival, growth, reproduction, and mastery. Adaptive responses in forms of behavior contribute to this goal or purpose. Health is a reflection of adaptation, the process of interaction between the person and the environment. In her earlier writings, she viewed health as a continuum from peak wellness or highest level of health to extreme poor health and death. Her later views focused more on health as a process in which health and illness can exist together in the person's total life dimension. When humans are able to use adaptive mechanisms affectively, health is maintained or achieved. It is when these adaptive mechanisms are ineffective or fail when illness or disease ensues.[4,12]

Martha Rogers: Unitary Human Beings (1970)

The theory of Unitary Human Beings by Martha Rogers emerged out of her strong liberal arts and science background. The knowledge base of her theory is rooted in multiple disciplines such as anthropology, psychology, sociology, astronomy, religion, philosophy, history, biology, physics, mathematics, and literature. This model of unitary human beings was first published in 1970 and represents a synthesis of her global thinking. The central components of the Rogerian model are unitary human beings and the environment. The model links the energy fields of the **environment** as an integral part of the human being and vice versa. The influences of Einstein's theory of relativity and general system theory introduced by von Bertalanffy are evident in the theory. This model was developed against the backdrop of new knowledge and information about the traditional meanings of homeostasis, steady state, adaptation, and equilibrium.[6]

The Rogers' Unitary Being Model rests on four basic foundations: 1) energy field, 2) a universe of open systems, 3) pattern, and 4) four dimensionality. It postulates that human beings are dynamic energy fields that are integral parts of the **environment** which is also an energy field. Human beings continuously exchange matter and energy with one another, giving rise to the concept of openness. It views the universe as composing of open systems with energy fields that are infinite, open, and integral with one another. Both the human being and the environment are energy fields. The distinguishing characteristic of an energy field is a pattern and perceived as a single wave. Each human field pattern is unique to the individual and is an integral part of the environmental field. This human being-environment relationship is manifested through **behaviors,** qualities, and unique individual characteristics. The human energy field, as an integral part of the environmental energy field, is a unified whole and more than the sum total of his individual parts.

To Rogers, **health** is a value term defined by the culture or individual. Health and illness are manifestations of pattern and these could be high value (maximum health) or low value (illness). The life of human beings are manifested in the life process which indicates the degree to which the individual achieves maximum health according to some value systems. Nursing's purpose is to promote health and well-being of all people in the world in which they live. This includes the **environment** that affects the individual's life processes. Martha Rogers' view that nursing encompasses the totality of human beings and their environments within a pan— dimensional universe of **open systems** opens the door to a new identity of nursing as a science with her science-based model of Unitary Human Beings.

Margaret Newman: Model of Health (1978)

Newman first presented her theory of health in 1978 wherein she identified her major concept of health as an "expanding consciousness".[6] Consciousness refers to person, client, individual, or human beings, and used interchangeably. Persons, which she expanded to include family and community, are centers of consciousness and part of the overall pattern of expanding consciousness.[13] She derives her theory from many philosophical sources and was influenced by such nursing theorists as Rogers and Johnson.[6] The basic concepts of her theory—movement, space, time and consciousness, were underpinnings of her model. Her life experiences gave a more personal meaning to her concept of **illness** and **health** which led to her recognition of pattern in each person's life. Pattern is what gives individuality to a person. Characteristics of pattern include movement, diversity, and rhythm.

In Newman's view, the phenomena of health is the manifestation of that evolving pattern. Health is regarded as an evolving pattern of the person and the environment. Her view of health encompasses both disease and nondisease. Disease is a manifestation of the pattern of health. This was based on the philosophical assumption of Hagel's "fusion of opposites".[6] Health and disease, although opposite states, are meaningful manifestations of the pattern of the whole. Expanding consciousness is an ongoing process manifested by patterns of the whole. The expansion of consciousness defines what life is about, and therefore, also defines health. The last stage of absolute consciousness is when contrasting concepts and opposites are fused and reconciled to comprise the whole. She applied her concepts of space, time, and movement in terms of client situations where people move through space and time in an ever-expanding consciousness. The person is the center of consciousness intersected by movement, time, and space and varies from person to person, place to place or time to time.

The concept of environment, although not explicitly defined, is referred to as beyond the scope of consciousness but constitutes the larger pattern of the whole. The interaction between the person and environment is crucial to the creation of the pattern configuration for each individual. An assumption of this theory is that the universe-environment is composed of matter. Patterns of this person-environment interaction evolve to higher levels of consciousness for the self.

Nurses are viewed as part of the process of expanding consciousness of the individual by developing a relationship with clients at important points in their lives, such as during illness or disability. They participate in the client's life process and expanding consciousness. Nurse and client are seen as partners in this process. They also assist the client in recognizing their own patterns of interacting with the environment. The process of pattern recognition on a particular client involves holistic observations of the person-environment behaviors that reflect a particular pattern of the whole for each person.

Madeleine Leininger: Culture Care: Diversity and Universality Theory (1991)

Leininger's theory of Culture Care is derived from the field of anthropology and nursing. In her studies of culture and actually living with the indigenous people of New Guinea, she developed a greater understanding of the role of **culture** in health practices. It was in the 1950's and 1960's that Leininger was able to identify areas common to anthropology and nursing and began to formulate transcultural concepts. This laid the foundation for developing her Transcultural Care theory and culturally based health care. She was the first professional nurse to obtain a doctoral degree in anthropology. She has studied as many as 14 major cultures and has had experience in many other cultures. Her extensive background in cultures of many people gave her a unique perspective in developing greater understanding of the relevance of culture in caring for people from diverse backgrounds. Her Theory of Culture Care is now widely recognized throughout the world as an essential component to modern health care. She changed and enlarged the approach to nursing care to include the cultural components in the **holistic** care of people in any setting. In Leininger's view, culture is the broadest approach to understanding people. Cultural knowledge has become an imperative in nursing education and practice. This transcultural component, Leininger believes, is what distinguishes nursing from other disciplines.

The theory of Culture Care is considered a middle-range theory and includes many relevant terms and definitions[6] such as culture, care, cultural care, cultural care universality, cultural care diversity, worldview, environmental context, health, cultural congruence, cultural and social structure dimensions, among others. Culture is the learned, shared, and transmitted values, beliefs, norms, and lifeway of a particular group that guides their thinking, decisions and actions in patterned ways. Care refers to those behaviors towards others that are meant to mitigate or improve human conditions through assisting, supporting and enabling actions. Cultural care are values, beliefs and patterns of living learned and transmitted within the culture that assist, support, facilitate, or enable another individual or group to maintain their **well-being** and **health**, to improve their human conditions, or deal with illness, disability, or death. Cultural care universality refers to those patterns of behavior, values, symbols, or meanings that are common, similar or dominant in many cultures which assist, support, or enable individuals from different cultures. Health is defined by Leininger as a state of well-being that is culturally defined, valued, practiced and reflects the ability of individuals or groups to perform activities in their daily lives reflecting their culture. The nurse provides interventions to clients of varied cultures based on the following:[5] 1. culture care preservation and maintenance, 2. culture care accommodation, negotiation, or both, and 3. culture care restructuring and repatterning.

Jean Watson: Philosophy and Science of Caring

Jean Watson's philosophy centered around the concept of **caring**. In Watson's view, caring is the essence of nursing practice. Her philosophy is relevant to the concept of balance because of its focus on the caring approach in nursing practice, an approach that brought new dimensions to the nurse-patient relationship. Watson's theory is composed of 10 carative factors which serve as her philosophical foundation for the science of caring and provide specific direction for nursing actions. These are:[6]

1. Formation of a humanistic-altruistic system of values
2. Instillation of faith-hope
3. Cultivation of sensitivity to self and to others
4. Development of a helping-trust relationship
5. Promotion and acceptance of the expression of positive and negative feelings
6. Systematic use of the scientific problem-solving method for decision-making
7. Promotion of interpersonal teaching-learning
8. Provision for supportive, protective, and corrective mental, physical, sociocultural, and spiritual environment
9. Assistance with gratification of human needs
10. Allowance for existential, phenomenological forces

Noting that the art of caring was gradually losing emphasis in the healthcare system, Watson sought to revitalize this more humanistic approach. Watson views health as the **unity** and **harmony** between mind, body, and soul. Nursing's goal is to help the person achieve this higher degree of harmony.

COMMON ELEMENTS OF BALANCE IN SELECTED NURSING THEORIES

The following summarizes the common elements of balance found in the nursing theories cited:

Theorist	Theory/Model	Balance Elements
Florence Nightingale	Environment	Environmental effects on health and illness
Betty Neuman	Systems Model	Environments, open systems, survival, stress harmony and balance, adaptation, needs
Dorothy Johnson	Behavioral System Model	Behavior, equilibrium, stability, adaptations, balance, harmony, system
Sister Callista Roy	Adaptation Model	Adaptation, environment, behaviors, health, adaptive system, coping mechanisms
Martha Rogers	Unitary Human Beings	Environment, behaviors, health, open systems
Margaret Newman	Model of Health	Health, illness, environment
Madeleine Leininger	Culture Care	Culture, well-being, health, holistic
Jean Watson	Caring	Harmony within mind, body, and soul

It is evident that there are commonalties of some elements in the view of these theorists. Their philosophical and theoretical foundations did not spring from a vacuum. They were drawn from concepts used in other disciplines and scientific approaches. Nursing practice in today's world requires a strong scientific base. The discipline of nursing cannot stand alone without the foundation drawn from other disciplines such the physical, social, and behavioral sciences. The concept of balance and its elements provide known evidence of this pool of knowledge that nursing can draw from. The core elements of balance such as homeostasis, equilibrium, adaptation, needs and health/wellness are abundant in literatures in most disciplines. Other related concepts such as evolution, behavior, stability, harmony, systems, environments, culture, personality, family and social systems are all part of the universality of balance. No one concept is more all-encompassing and universal so far in this stage of development of nursing science.

The most frequently recurring element identified was the environment, a core element in the concept of balance. Although the distinction between the internal environment and the outside environment may not necessarily be explicit in all of the theories, the recognition of the central role of this concept is quite evident. Florence Nightingale for instance, made environment as the most important element that affects people's health and causes illness in her view. This philosophy laid the foundation for future views of other theorists in the search for improvement of nursing practice and the science of nursing. The environment is also a major concept in the theories of Betty Neuman, Sister Callista Roy, Martha Rogers, and Margaret Newman. Roy in particular, considers the environment as constantly changing and stimulates the person to make adaptive responses. These responses are evidenced by behavior that are measurable, describable, and observable. In Dorothy Johnson's Behavioral System Model, the person is a behavioral system that seeks stability and balance by making adaptations and adjustments to the environment.

Health and illness, two dichotomous aspects of balance, are imbedded in these selected nursing theories, whether or not they are specifically defined. These are usually associated with nursing's role of caring for individuals in health and in sickness. Florence Nightingale wrote of the goal of nurses as facilitating the body's reparative processes by environmental manipulation, suggesting that these interventions promote health and prevent illness. Rogers views the role of nursing as maintaining and promoting health, preventing illness, and caring for the 'Unitary human beings" through the humanistic science of nursing. Roy views people as adaptive systems; the goal of nursing is to help people adapt to physiologic and psychosocial changes during health and illness. Leininger takes the broad view that the definition of health and health beliefs differ among various cultures and should be considered as part of culture care.

Behavior involves movement and a universal characteristic of all living human beings. Behavior drives change in response to stimuli, whatever the stimuli may be. Behavior is necessarily involved in all aspects of life. These nursing theories and concepts provide snapshots of their view of human behavior—both that of the client's or of the nurse. These theorists see human behavior through the lens of their individual perspectives against philosophical and theoretical influences from other disciplines. Roy, Neuman, Johnson, and Rogers view human behaviors as a reflection of the dynamic interaction between man and the environment. Their models are derived from system theory developed by other disciplines. Client behaviors are used as measures of the state of health or illness, basis for observation and evaluation of effectiveness of interventions, or to determine the person's cultural perspectives. Behavior is viewed as movements within an open system that receives input (stimuli) and produces output (behavior).

The more direct use of the concept of balance is not found in more explicit terms in these selected theories. Balance as a core concept is not used as a cohesive framework but as part of the model or philosophy of these theories. Nursing's role in health and illness does not delve more into the depth of nurses' involvement in the preservation and protection of the life of human beings, thereby ensuring their survival. Roy's Adaptation model comes fairly close to this balance framework. Drawn from the previous works of Harry Helson in psychophysics and Rapoport's system definition,[6] Roy developed the concept of the person as an adaptive system. The very concept of adaptation involves the ability of human beings and other life forms on this planet to survive and thrive within their environment. If human beings depend on their ability to adapt, then it stands to reason that this mechanism is one of the most important means for survival. Nursing is a discipline that supports, maintains, restores and assists clients in preserving their health and wellbeing. It must be engaged in activities that preserve human survival through helping clients in their adaptive responses to stimuli affecting them.

Neuman's System theory and Dorothy Johnson' Behavioral System Model also touch on an important concept of balance: the open system. Further reinforced by Roy's adaptive systems, the open system lends more strength to the idea that man is part of, or functions within an open system. As the term suggests, an open system is one that is, not only open to outside stimuli (input), but also responds accordingly through behaviors. In human beings, there are also influences or stimuli coming from within the body itself—whether created physiologically, or mentally through thought processes, such as emotions, beliefs and attitudes. These bits of stimuli can also generate physiological reactions, such as the effects of perceived stress by the individual. Human beings are always in dynamic interaction with their environment. This interaction is conceived as an open system because the boundaries between the internal and external environments cannot necessarily be rigid. A porous or permeable boundary has to exist for stimuli to go through and exit from, to enable the human being to survive and thrive.

Another important element of balance is equilibrium, a term not often found in nursing theories. Dorothy Johnson's Behavioral System Model uses equilibrium as one of its important concepts. She views the person as a behavioral system that seeks stability and balance with his or her environment through adaptations and adjustments. Equilibrium is achieved when a state of harmony exists between the individual and the environment. Stresses disrupt this equilibrium. Failure to use adaptive processes to maintain equilibrium causes instability, which leads to illness. The concepts of balance and imbalance are applied although not succinctly stated. Behavioral outcomes are the manifestations of this process which nurses can observe and influence through nursing interventions.

The role of culture in psychosocial balance is a new approach advanced by Madeleine Leininger in her Culture Care Model. As the discipline of nursing spread all over the world and became a global profession, it became apparent that a new approach to caring for patients coming from various cultural backgrounds is imperative. The influence of culture on beliefs, attitudes and practices was an important element of behavior. The discipline of sociology lent more credence to this view in that individuals are viewed as part of the community and society of which they are part. Health beliefs and practices affect outcomes. Treatments and interventions that are congruent with people's cultural beliefs are more likely to bring about the desired outcomes that nursing is aiming for. Spiritual beliefs that have been passed on from generation to generation through the vehicle of culture have provided emotional stability and anchor to people who have to deal with the misfortunes of life.

Thus, it becomes apparent that the concept of balance can be directly applied to the practice of nursing. The universality of the concept of balance is consistent with the goals of nursing: to provide care that aims to promote, restore, and maintain health and well-being of individuals, families and communities. Health as central to the nursing discipline is anchored on the respect for life, its protection and preservation through the actions of the nurse. Understanding the roots of survival and the elements that are necessary for it becomes crucial to the nurse's understanding of her own place in the larger scheme of the universe.

Jean Watson's Theory of Caring can be incorporated into a nursing model that emphasizes the humanistic approach of caring for the whole person—mind, body, and soul. This can be demonstrated through interpersonal relationships with clients in the nursing process. The Caring Theory emphasizes use of the scientific problem-solving approach in the nursing process as well as meeting the needs of clients in the biophysical and psychosocial realms—all based on Maslow's Hierarchy of Needs and further developed in the Behavior Pyramid. By using caring principles, balance-seeking behaviors can be better achieved.

KEY CONCEPTS:

• •

1. The core pillars of balance/imbalance—homeostasis, adaptation, equilibrium, needs, and health—as well as its related concepts of behavior, environment, culture, and systems, are all within the holistic view of the nursing profession. Balance is a concept that governs all areas of human existence.

2. Nursing evolved from its early beginnings along with the medical profession but has taken another direction and defined itself as a different field through the efforts of many nursing leaders.

3. Nursing has developed a unique body of knowledge based on nursing theories and borne by research which all contributed to its professional development. Theories are the most concrete components of nursing that were formulated to guide its practice.

4. The domain of nursing includes the concepts of person, environment, health, and nursing. These concepts provide the structure to the discipline and define its theoretical boundaries. A metaparadigm identifies the specific phenomena related to the discipline; a paradigm is a particular viewpoint or way of thinking within the discipline. A view of balance as a paradigm needs to be further explored and developed.

5. The care of human beings is the focus of nursing and this basic philosophy is found in nursing theories. The concept of balance provides the framework for caring for all human beings. It is directly concerned with supporting survival and meeting basic needs essential for health.

6. The works of several authors that support the concept of balance in caring for people are mentioned. These authors are: Florence Nightingale (Environment theory), Betty Neuman (Systems Model), Dorothy Johnson (Behavioral System), Sister Callista Roy (Adaptation Model), Martha Rogers (Unitary Human Beings), Margaret Newman (Model of Health), Medeleine Leininger (Culture Care), and Jean Watson (Caring). Common elements of balance were identified in these theories.

7. The role of culture in caring for culturally diverse populations is a relatively recent approach advanced by Madeleine Leininger. Recognition of the centrality of culture in nursing care has spread around the world. Culture is part of the external environment of balance that has influenced human behavior, attitudes, and beliefs that impact health behaviors.

8. The universality of the concept of balance is consistent with the goals of nursing. Understanding the roots of survival and the elements necessary to preserve, restore, promote, and maintain health and well-being are crucial to professional nursing practice.

CHAPTER 7: THEORETICAL UNDERPINNINGS IN NURSING

REFERENCES

1. Nightingale, Florence. (1859). Notes in Nursing. Reprinted in *Notes on Nursing: What it is and What it is not*. Foreword by V. Dunbar, preface by Margaret Dolan (1969). New York. Dover Publications, Inc.
2. The Florence Nightingale Pledge. http://www.truthaboutnursing.org/press/pioneers/nightingale_pledge.html. (retrieved 1/18/2013.
3. History of Medicine-Wikipedia, the free encyclopedia. http://en.wikipedia.org/wiki/history_of_medicine. (retrieved 1/18/2013).
4. Daniels, R., Grendell, R.N., and Wilkins, F.R.2010. *Nursing Fundamentals: Caring and Clinical Decision Making (2ⁿᵈ ed.)* Clifton Park, NY. Delmar.
5. Potter, P.A. and Perry, A.G. 2005. *Fundamentals of Nursing (6ᵗʰ ed.)* St. Louis, Missouri. Mosby, Inc.
6. Tomey, A. M. and Alligood, M.R. 2002. *Nursing Theorists and their Work* (5ᵗʰ ed.) St. Louis, Missouri. Mosby, Inc.
7. Mosby's *Dictionary of Medicine, Nursing & Health Professions (7ᵗʰ ed.)* 2006. St. Louis, Missouri. Mosby Elsevier.
8. What is Systems Theory? http://pespmc1.vub.ac.be/SYSTHEOR.html. (retrieved 1/24/2013).
9. Freese, B.T. 2002. *"Betty Neuman: Systems Model"*. in Tomey, A.M. and Alligood, M.R. *Nursing Theorists and their Work (5ᵗʰ ed.)* St. Louis, Missouri. Mosby, Inc.
10. Roy, C. 1984. *Introduction to Nursing: An Adaptation Model (2ⁿᵈ ed.)* Englewood Cliffs, NJ. Prentice Hall.
11. Roy, C. & Andrews, H.A. 1991. *The Roy Adaptation Model: The Definitive Statement.* Norwalk, CT. Appleton & Lange.
12. Phillips, K.D. 2002. "Sister Callista Roy: Adaptation Model". In Tomey, A.M. and Alligood, M.R. *Nursing Theorists and their Work (5ᵗʰ ed.)* St. Louis, Missouri. Mosby, Inc.
13. Witucki, J.M. 2002. "Margaret Newman: Model of Health". in Tomey, A.M. and Alligood, M.R. *Nursing Theorists and their Work (5ᵗʰ ed.)* St. Louis, Missouri. Mosby, Inc.

Chapter 8

THE NURSING PROCESS BALANCE MODEL

"A new vision of development is emerging. Development is becoming a people-centered process, whose ultimate goal must be the improvement of the human condition."
—Boutros Boutros-Ghali (former UN Secretary-General)

Improvement of the human condition is a concern not just of international leaders but also that of nursing. Nursing is a profession that has been concerned with improving the health of people, helping people, and advocating for people. The clients in nursing are not just individuals, but also families and communities. The multi-disciplinary, holistic approach to nursing care has made nursing a very unique profession. It has no boundaries—it treats people regardless of race, gender, religion, or culture. Nursing can be found where there are people. As long as a human life exists, nursing does its part to save it, restore its health, preserve its dignity, and help enable individuals to achieve their fullest potential. As long as humans strive to seek balance in their lives but fail to do so, nursing helps in its restoration. If humans engage in behaviors that jeopardize lives and safety, nursing plays a part in modifying that behavior. The process used by nurses and at the core of its professional practice is the **nursing process.**

Traditional nursing process provides a framework for professional nursing practice through steps that are logical, systematic, holistic, and client-centered. It uses the skills of the nurse in critical thinking, clinical decision-making, communication, and interpersonal relations based on knowledge, educational preparation, experience, research evidence, and technological know-how. The modern professional nurse has the tools needed to provide the best of care. And yet, these tools can still be constantly improved. Frames of references can change and paradigms can shift over time, as new ways of thinking evolve and as humans evolve. There is a need for a more universal framework and a frame of reference that has broad acceptance and application in the human fields of endeavor. This framework is provided by the nursing process approach which has gained universal acceptance in the profession.

OVERVIEW OF THE TRADITIONAL NURSING PROCESS

The nursing process is an organizing framework in nursing that involves the use of systematic and logical steps to achieve the goal of nursing: the provision of professional and quality nursing care. It is what differentiates nursing practice from that of physicians and other health care professionals. Through the use of an individualized approach to patient care, it enables the nurse to provide a unique, timely, and holistic approach for each client. Nursing has evolved into a science-based profession where nursing actions are based on rationale. It utilizes client data from various sources in order to arrive at an identification of client problems. By utilizing its broad base of knowledge in the various sciences, nursing has been able to keep in lock-step with the other professions. It involves critical thinking, problem—solving, and decision-making through the following steps in the nursing process: [1,2]

1. Assessment
2. Nursing diagnosis
3. Planning and outcome identification
4. Implementation
5. Evaluation

Assessment

Assessment is the first step in the nursing process which requires deliberate and systematic collection of data to determine the patient's current health status, past health history, functional level, socio-cultural determinants, and important beliefs or influences that impinge on the patient's present state of health. The purpose of assessment is to establish a **data base** about the patient which contributes to the patient/client health problems and his/her responses to these problems. It is important to obtain accurate and verifiable data from various sources—both primary and secondary. **Primary** sources of data are those obtained directly from the client, whether it is described, measured, or observed. **Secondary** sources are those obtained from medical records, other health professionals, family, friends, or significant others.

Primary data that are directly reported by the patient are called **subjective data,** which includes the patient's description of their symptoms, feelings, and perceptions relevant to their condition. Those that are obtained from the client through the use of direct observation or instruments are called **objective data.** Measurement of objective data should be based on standardized measures, such as a thermometer for temperature, a weighing scale for weight, a measuring cup for amount of liquid such as urine, a glucometer to determine fingerstick blood sugar, or a measuring tape to measure abdominal girth or wound size. The stethoscope has become an important tool for the nurse to perform objective physical assessment by listening to breath sounds, abdominal sounds, heart sounds, and obtaining blood pressure. Methods of physical assessment such as inspection, auscultation, palpation, and percussion are utilized in modern nursing practice. These techniques of data—gathering require the clinical skills and expertise of the professional nurse. It is important for the nurse to report and document these findings accurately and concisely based on objective measures.

Secondary data sources are those that pertain to, but not directly obtained from the client, such as the client medical records, other health professionals such as the doctor or other nurses, the patient's family, and others who have knowledge about the client. However, for patients who are unable to verbalize or do not have the capacity for whatever reason, such as infants and children, unconscious, critically ill, mentally handicapped, or those with reduced cognitive functions, the family may be the primary source of information. The members of the health care team who had direct contact with the patient /client, such as the primary physician or specialists, dieticians, social workers, respiratory therapists, or physical therapists, also serve as important sources of information. Medical records provide important client information, especially reports of diagnostic tests and procedures such as laboratory tests, radiologic studies, and diagnostic procedures. All these contribute towards piecing together a comprehensive picture of the health status of the patient.

Once data are gathered and organized, a **data base** is formed which provides the basis for analyzing the client's health problems and need for health and nursing services. By **clustering data**, a pattern or patterns begin to emerge to identify the client's problems. It is important to prioritize the client's problems to address problems or needs that have to be addressed first—from the most life-threatening to the least but can have long-term effects on patient outcomes. Failure to address life-threatening situations and not acting upon this assessment with utmost expediency can endanger the patient's life. A trained nurse can easily identify an emergency situation whereas a less experienced nurse may not. This is where clinical expertise and experience play a major role in making clinical judgments. Application of critical thinking and problem-solving skills are necessary to arrive at the appropriate identification of the patient's problems.

Nursing Diagnosis

Nursing Diagnosis is a clinical judgment about individual, family, or community responses to actual and potential health problems or life processes which provide the basis for the selection of nursing interventions to achieve outcomes for which the nurse has accountability (NANDA International, 2005).[3] This second step in the nursing process is the result of analysis of data obtained from and about the patient from various sources. It describes the patient's actual or potential **response to a health problem** which the nurse, by virtue of her or his professional license is legally responsible to treat or resolve. Patient responses to health problems are determined by analyzing and interpreting data that have been gathered, clustered and prioritized. These responses are in terms of behavioral manifestations that fall within or outside the norm. Age-specific factors are also considered in that normal values in one age group differ from other age groups. For instance, normal values in infants are quite different from that of an elderly client. Selection of appropriate nursing diagnoses will lead to appropriate nursing interventions.

Nursing diagnosis marks the divergence between nursing practice and medical practice. A **medical diagnosis** is the identification of the cause of disease conditions or illness by the use of combined physical examination, patient interview, laboratory tests, review of the patient's medical records, knowledge of the cause of observed signs and symptoms, and differential elimination of similar possible cause.[4] Its goal is the identification, treatment, and cure of the disease or pathological process. Both use patient data from various sources and both use evidence and analytical reasoning to arrive at a diagnosis. However, medical diagnosis is centered on the disease process and its treatment through medications, invasive and non-invasive therapies, surgery, and other treatment modalities following the practices of Western medicine. Nursing diagnosis on the other hand, is a clinical judgment about the client's **response** to health care problems based on an analysis of data. A nurse cannot independently treat a medical diagnosis such as diabetes or congestive heart failure. However, the nurse can manage the medications, activity, and diet of the patient based on his or her response to the treatment ordered by the physician. Problems that require combined nursing and medical interventions are called **collaborative problems**. This is where a true partnership between the physician and the nurse takes place.

The formulation of nursing diagnoses has been standardized by the North American Nursing Diagnosis Association International (**NANDA-I**) to have a common language that can be used by nurses all over the world. It identified three types of nursing diagnoses: actual diagnoses, risk diagnoses, and wellness diagnoses. An **actual nursing diagnosis** describes human conditions or responses that exist in an individual, family, or community supported by sufficient assessment data that the problem actually exists. **A risk diagnosis** describes responses to health conditions or processes that have a high likelihood of developing in a vulnerable individual, family, or community. There are available data that support the risk or vulnerability of the client. It includes risk factors such as environmental, physiological, psychological, genetic, or chemical element. **Wellness diagnosis** describes the client's readiness for a higher level of health. The nurse incorporates the client's strengths and support systems into the plan of care and the expected outcome directed at an enhanced state of health.

Nursing diagnostic statements can have one, two, or three parts.[5] The two-part format is the more simple way of stating the nursing diagnosis without undue oversimplification. The **diagnostic label** is the name of the nursing diagnosis as derived from assessment data and approved by NANDA International. Descriptive terms such as impaired, compromised, decreased, delayed, or ineffective provide additional meaning and clarification of the condition. **Related factors** are conditions or causative factor (etiology) associated with the patient's actual or potential response to a health problem. These are factors that can be changed by using appropriate nursing interventions. This is where nursing interventions can change client responses to their health problems. By understanding the underlying cause or etiology, behavioral responses can be altered to result in positive outcomes for the client. An example of a two-part nursing diagnosis is: *activity intolerance* (diagnostic label) *related to generalized body weakness* (etiology or cause). Use of related factors requires critical thinking analysis of assessment data to individualize the nursing diagnosis and determine nursing interventions appropriate for the patient. Various references are available to understand further the formulation of the nursing diagnosis based on the NANDA International classification.[6,7] There are non-NANDA-approved diagnoses which are still the subject of debate among various educational and service institutions.

Planning

Planning, the third step in nursing process includes at least four basic steps: *goal-setting, determining outcomes, establishing priorities,* and selection of *interventions* to meet the desired patient goals. It is necessary for the nurse to establish a *rationale* for nursing interventions formulated. This is where evidence-based practice is implemented utilizing knowledge from research in nursing and related professions. Goals are specific targets that nurses aim to reach in order to realize desired outcomes. Goals and expected outcomes have to be patient-centered, observable, measurable, time-limited, and realistic. They reflect the change in patient behavior and responses as a result of nursing interventions. These are not the nurses' personal goals but rather the patient's desired behavioral outcomes. It has to be stated as such in order to make these patient-centered goals clear to everyone in the health care team. Most of all, the client and his or her family need to be involved in setting realistic goals.

Priority-setting involves ranking nursing diagnoses in their order of importance. Priorities can be classified as high, intermediate, or low. Problems that directly impact survival need to be addressed immediately and has the highest priority. For example, a patient in respiratory distress needs immediate attention as failure to do so will mean death for the client. Although physiologic needs often have the highest priority, psychological or safety needs sometimes take a higher priority. A patient in immediate danger of falling out of bed should be given the highest priority over the physiologic need for water or nutrition.

Planning also involves identification of appropriate **nursing interventions** that are within the scope of practice of the nurse. Nursing interventions should to be client-centered and individualized to meet the patient's established goals and outcomes. Selection of nursing interventions are based on the following competence of the nurse: 1) must have the knowledge of the scientific rationale for the interventions, 2) possess the necessary physical, technical, and interpersonal skills to perform the interventions (or able to delegate these to appropriate personnel), 3) able to function within the health care setting where client care is provided, as well as utilize available resources in that setting. A **written plan of care** is generally used by nurses in health care settings and communicated to the members of the health care team. It is a tool that enhances communication, facilitates continuity of care, and ensures the consistency of nursing interventions to meet identified goals.

Implementation

Implementation is the phase in the nursing process where actual performance of nursing actions are carried out based on problems identified via assessment, nursing diagnosis, and goal-setting. It involves the provision of care based on a plan through the performance of specific **nursing interventions**. A nursing intervention is an act of the nurse based on clinical judgment, knowledge, and skills to achieve desired patient outcomes.[8] Interventions are provided directly or indirectly to the nurse's clients—individuals, families, and community— using a caring approach. **Direct interventions** are those actions such as treatments, medications, positioning, wound care, etc. that are provided by the nurse directly to the patient. The nursing skills required to carry out appropriate implementation of interventions include cognitive, psychomotor, and interpersonal skills. **Indirect interventions** are those for which the nurse is still responsible but are provided by others on behalf of the patient under the supervision of the nurse. Examples are tasks such as taking vital signs or bathing done by assistive personnel who have the skills to perform the delegated tasks. It is expected that nursing interventions are provided with the use of critical thinking and constant reassessment of the patient before, during, and after interventions to determine the effects of these actions on patient responses. Safety and patient comfort are always factors that need to be taken into consideration in collaboration with the patient and their family. Patient responses to treatment should always be recorded accurately and concisely. Interventions are carried out by the nurse with a scientific rationale in mind and with a caring heart.

Evaluation

Evaluation is the fifth phase in the nursing process that involves determination of whether the interventions were able to produce the outcomes identified in patient care goals. Desired outcomes may not be immediately met, such as the effects on healing in wound care after one treatment. In this case, the effect of such treatment or treatments needs to be evaluated over time. Or, the outcome may be observed over a short period of time, such as the effect on patient comfort after changing the patient's position. For instance, activity tolerance could be immediately determined by ambulating the patient according to the level set as part of the goals. Evaluation is done on an ongoing basis through assessment and reassessment of the patient matched against the goals set for the specific individual. As in the other phases of the nursing process, critical thinking is used to determine the answers to some questions used in evaluating patient progress. Some of these questions are: How do I determine if the interventions were effective? If the patient was not able to achieve the desired goals, what can be done differently to make it more effective? What other data are needed to identify the reason or reasons for persistence of the problem? Are there other factors that have not been considered in determining the patient's problems? Would it require the assistance of other personnel? Does the patient have a thorough understanding of the goals and has the capacity to cooperate?

It is important to remember that the patient is also part of the team. Engaging the patient's cooperation and providing motivations to participate in his or her own care enable patients to feel that they are part of their own goals to achieve well-being and healing. The nurse also needs to do some introspection and self-evaluation to look at her own attitude and actions that may affect the nurse-patient interaction. It is helpful to discuss the patient's plan of care with other members of the health care team, and the family if possible, to find better solutions to persistent and unresolved problems. Following reassessment of data and team conference with other players involved in the patient's care, another plan of care may have to be developed and new goals may need to be identified that are more realistic and do-able for the patient. Consistently incorporating the process of evaluation in all aspects of client care will help in implementing the nursing process more effectively to achieve desired patient outcomes.

THE NURSING PROCESS BALANCE MODEL

Models in nursing are developed to provide a framework for practice. By using balance as an approach in the development of a comprehensive model of nursing practice, a new dimension is opened. Using the nursing process as a framework for determining the client's health status, essentially getting a clearer picture of the client's state of balance, underscores the role of the nurse in health care. Using a scientific approach, astute data-gathering and critical thinking, the client's response to health problems can be identified. Various indicators, both qualitative and quantitative can be used in data-gathering. The indicators are behavioral measures of the degree of balance and imbalance of the client, hence, an indication of his/her state of health. The nursing process also uses as much data as possible about the client—their health behaviors, risk behaviors, influencing factors in the external environment, and internal factors affecting the client's behavior. By using a health-illness balance continuum developed in the previous chapter, a comprehensive approach of the nursing process is developed.

Overview and Rationale

A Nursing Process Balance Model hereby proposed is one that incorporates the nursing process and the concept of balance with its elements of equilibrium, homeostasis, adaptation, needs, and health within the internal and external environments, into a more comprehensive approach to nursing practice. Client behavior and communication between the nurse and the client are key components of this model. The goal of nursing process used in the nurse-patient interaction is modifying or changing the client behavior into balance-seeking behaviors within their realms of behavior in the Behavior Pyramid. Balance at each realm is determined by the individual himself and should be used by the nurse as the frame of reference for interventions. As we know, behaviors are actions or movements that are observable, describable and measurable. Behaviors are the outputs in the human system functioning within the health-illness continuum. These behaviors become the feedback to the nurse to evaluate the effectiveness of nursing interventions.

The nurse and client are both products of their internal and external environments and the influence of balance elements. They share basic commonalities: their human traits composed of physical, psychological, mental, emotional, and biologic characteristics. Both are social beings within their individual family unit, community and society. Both are subject to the influences of nature and its elements. Their differences lie in the role that they play in the nurse-patient interaction. Nurses, by virtue of their training and educational background, are in a position to assist the client to modify imbalanced behaviors that brought them to the health care system. Nurses are able to intervene in life-threatening situations and restore clients to a better state of health. They are agents of caring and healing. The nursing process enables the nurse to help clients achieve health and balance.

The Nursing Process Balance model has principles that are based on solid foundations of the sciences. The basic elements of the balance—homeostasis, equilibrium, adaptation, needs, and health—concepts derived from existing sciences and universal knowledge that have been used for many generations. The discovery and development of these concepts are products of intellectual activities for thousands of years by human beings. Whether these are articulated in theories or written literature or not does not change the evidence that these elements have existed with life on the planet. For nurses, as keepers of the art of caring and healing, using the nursing process based on the concept of balance provides a coherent and universal approach, and a rationale for more comprehensive nursing care.

Nursing functions in the Model

Nurses can change client behavioral responses through three main functions: 1. restorative, 2. maintenance, and 3. preventive. These functions remain intact in the Nursing Process Balance Model. The only difference is the approach and focus of the nursing process which centers on the concept of achieving balance in the lives and health of the client. In this model, the approach is in *the emphasis on the assessment of the state of balance and identification of imbalances in the client's health status.*

Restorative function is aimed at directly moving the patient from a state of imbalance to a state of balance compatible with survival. For example, a patient in a state of dehydration due to poor fluid intake can be restored to a state of balance by providing fluids to meet the body's requirements. By ensuring that the patient is able to take enough fluids, either orally, or through intravenous infusions ordered by the physician, the state of fluid balance can be restored. Continued dehydration can endanger the survival of the patient. The behavioral response of the dehydrated patient can be observed and monitored through **objective and subjective indicators**. A dehydrated patient may have any or all of the following signs and symptoms: subjective: complains of feeling thirsty, lips and skin are dry; objective: poor skin turgor, flushed dry skin, dry mucous membranes, low blood pressure, rapid heart rate, poor urine output, and concentrated urine. A patient who has been restored to a state of fluid balance will present a different picture: skin and mucous membranes more hydrated, improved skin turgor, vital signs are normal, improved urine output and less concentrated. The client's behavioral response to the state of imbalance was reversed, thus presenting a different clinical picture than that prior to nursing and medical interventions. It is also worthy to note that the role of the nurse as an educator is always part of the nursing process. Educating patients is one way of improving their coping skills. Providing information to clients on the importance of adequate fluid intake, recognizing signs of dehydration, and actions they can independently do to prevent dehydration depending on the cause, are nursing interventions that the nurse can do independently as a professional nurse.

Once a state of balance is achieved, clients can be assisted to maintain this state of health. This is the **maintenance** function of the nurse and an important one. Majority of the population that nurses serve are healthy and maintaining health is an important aspect of healthcare. It is only when clients become ill or go into a state of uncompensated imbalances that they enter the healthcare system to be provided with medical care. Most of the time, this is when nurses come in contact with their patients. Unless the nurse works in the public health system, most nurses are employed in hospitals and sub-acute facilities where patients are provided institutionalized care. When patients are discharged from these hospitals, they return to their families and communities where they become part of the general population considered healthy. However, some fragile individuals such as the elderly, chronically ill, or disabled, are not able to sustain a certain level of wellness and end up going back to the hospital for medical care. It is within this health-illness continuum that nurses should aim to maintain the health of the general public. By assisting clients and their families to learn healthy and balance-seeking behaviors, the likelihood of their re-entering the healthcare system is decreased.

Prevention of imbalances need to be done in tandem with restoration and maintenance functions. Recognizing risk factors and eliminating or keeping these from affecting or influencing the client are the essence of prevention. This is the proactive approach to nursing care. Anticipation of actual and potential risks to the patient will help offset the negative effects of imbalance-producing factors. For example, environmental elements such as smoke, fumes, smog, radiation, toxic gases, contaminated water and food supplies, can potentially harm the health of entire populations. Short-term and long-term effects of these harmful elements can be seen from the imbalances that these produce on the body. Governmental regulations have been implemented by many nations around the world to protect their populations and prevent illness and disease. Besides eliminating the sources of these dangerous environmental elements, nurses can educate their clients on adopting health lifestyles and balance-seeking behaviors. Change in behavior needs to start with each individual. With the "one client at a time" approach, teaching can be individualized and the care for each client fashioned according to identified problems and needs.

STEPS IN THE NURSING PROCESS BALANCE MODEL

The steps in the Nursing Process Balance model follow the traditional nursing process with some important differences. The Nursing Process Balance model is based on the foundations of the balance concept and defines the outcomes of care in terms of restoration and maintenance of balance and the prevention of imbalances. In this model, the goal of nursing is modifying or changing human responses through balance-seeking behaviors. It aims to re-establish stability and equilibrium in the client, who has experienced instability by imbalances in their physical, physiological or psychosocial beings. All the factors that contributed to this imbalance need to be examined and data collected to determine the patient's level of response. Effective coping mechanisms need to be strengthened (maintained) while ineffective ones need to be changed (restored). Factors which pose a risk or threat to the state of balance of the patient should also be addressed to prevent imbalance (prevention). In these three areas, nursing can provide the appropriate interventions that will help move the patient from a state of illness to a state of wellness—a state where the patient is functioning at his or her optimal level of health. This is achieved by assisting clients to change behavioral responses from ineffective coping to effective coping that are balance seeking.

Assessment: using physiologic and psychosocial indicators

This is the first phase where data are collected using various methods and tools that are standardized and practiced in current health care settings. Assessment uses physiological and psychological **indicators of imbalance** using quantitative and qualitative data. **Quantitative data** include a physiologic systems assessment by surveying the functions of the various systems for signs and symptoms of imbalance. Laboratory tests and physical assessment can reveal these imbalances. The physiological systems survey should start with a **primary assessment** of the neurologic, respiratory, and cardiovascular systems or those basal life indicators that support life. Homeostatic mechanisms also need to be assessed via laboratory tests, such as electrolytes, blood count, and chemistry. **Secondary assessment** includes other systems that are also important in maintaining body function and balance. Any abnormality in the findings should be documented as an imbalance.

After gathering the primary and secondary physiologic data (prioritized according to the most important problems that need to be resolved immediately—survival needs to be addressed first), relevant psychosocial data should be gathered in order to assemble a comprehensive picture of the patient. Contributory information such as subjective complaints of the patient, mental health status, health history, family relationships, cultural health beliefs and practices, spirituality, stress factors, coping mechanisms, and knowledge level need to be assessed. In a world that is becoming more global and multi-cultural, it is essential that **cultural data** should be obtained which would assist in understanding patients' response to their illness. Understanding culturally-determined behavioral responses gives nurses a window to obtain a better insight of the patient's viewpoint. Spector believes in designing **culturally and linguistically appropriate** services that lead to improved health care outcomes, efficiency, and patient satisfaction . . . [9] A more individualized approach can be designed for the patient that takes a holistic approach.

In obtaining psychosocial data, the **Behavior Pyramid** can be used as a frame of reference for determining what psycho-social needs are operational and most important at that particular time for the patient. For instance, if the patient is at the level where his/her spiritual needs are important, nursing interventions should be geared towards supporting the patient's spiritual needs. Perhaps giving the patient the opportunity for spiritual meditation, prayers, or bringing in a spiritual advisor can help provide emotional support and inner strength. The physiological effects of meditation have been demonstrated, such as lowering of blood pressure, slowing of breathing and respirations, and relaxing of muscles. Research-based findings should be utilized as current information becomes available.

Nursing Diagnosis: Identification of imbalances

Nursing diagnosis is a statement that represents a clinical judgment of the patient's response to a health problem as determined by the nurse based on critical thinking and assessment data. In the Nursing Process Balance Model, the patient's response is a behavioral manifestation of balance or imbalance. These behavioral responses can be observed, described, and measured. Responses that don't contribute to maintaining physiological, psychological, emotional, intellectual, and physical balance serve to destabilize and create imbalances. Health care professionals like nurses and doctors aim to restore and maintain a certain degree of balance on their patients to keep them within the zone of equilibrium in the health-wellness continuum.

A nursing diagnosis is composed of a **diagnostic label** and the related factor. There are basically four categories of related factors:[10,5] pathophysiological (biological or psychological), treatment-related, situational (environmental or personal), and maturational. Related factors are those that contribute to or are associated with the problem. It is not necessarily the etiology. The **etiology,** or the cause of the nursing problem and part of the nursing diagnosis, is a condition that responds to nursing interventions.

A typical nursing diagnosis is a two-part statement describing the imbalance of the patient. This statement must be behaviorally stated to describe the nature of the imbalance. For example, a patient experiencing respiratory difficulty from chronic obstructive pulmonary disease (COPD) could have a nursing diagnosis of: *Ineffective breathing related to narrowing of airways and inadequate oxygenation.* These are derived from physiologic and physical responses observed and measured in the patient, such as the respiratory rate and oxygen saturation (physiologic), and use of accessory muscles of breathing, restlessness (physical), and subjective complaints, such the patient saying, "I have a hard time breathing". This patient is in a state of imbalance of the respiratory system which could affect the other systems if not addressed in a timely manner. Ineffective breathing is a behavioral response that the nurse, through nursing interventions based on sound scientific principles, can change to put the patient back into a state of balance. A state of balance is when the breathing becomes effective, i.e. respiratory rate normal, oxygen saturation within normal, less use of accessory muscles to do the work of breathing, patient able to assume a more comfortable lying position, and stating that "I can breathe better". The nurse cannot change the medical diagnosis; the patient still has COPD. But by being able to change the patient's behavioral responses, the patient is able to go back to a state of balance.

Another responsibility of nurses is to manage **collaborative problems**. Collaborative problems are physiologic complications that nurses monitor to detect an onset or change in patient status using both physician-prescribed and nursing-prescribed interventions to minimize complications or worsening of the condition. Collaborative problems are stated with the diagnostic label "Potential complication" at the beginning of the statement. Examples are: *Potential complication: cardiac failure; Potential complication: renal failure; Potential complication: hypovolemia.* All steps of the nursing process are still involved but with a different approach.[5] For nursing diagnoses, assessment involves data collection to identify actual or potential factors and problems are identified. In collaborative problems, the focus is on determining physiologic stability or risk for instability. In the Nursing Process Balance Model, both nursing diagnoses and collaborative problems are indications of imbalances for patients. The goal of their interventions is to correct the imbalance and restore balance, or prevent further imbalances.

Planning: goal-setting, outcome identification, and nursing interventions

Planning is the third part of the nursing process and involves three aspects: goal-setting, outcome identification, and prescribing nursing interventions. A goal is a specific behavioral response that reflects the highest level of balance. Patient-centered goals reflect the optimum state of balance that the patient can possibly achieve given the specific situation of the patient. The most desirable goal should be the state of balance within the Zone of Equilibrium. Some patients may not be able to fully achieve this goal during a particular time. However, this should still remain as a long-term goal if at all possible. Goals could be **short-term** and **long-term**. Each goal should be time-limited, the time frame dependent on the nature of the problem, cause of the problem, ability of the patient, availability of resources and sometimes family support. The patient and the family should be involved in goal-setting so that these are mutually understood and accepted. When patients start to regain stability and balance, these goals become more and more acceptable to them.

Expected outcomes are specific changes in the patient's status that the nurse would like to see as a result of nursing interventions. It is a specific measurable change in patient status that is expected to occur in response to care provided by the nurse. This expectation is measured in terms of the goals of care. The goal of nursing care is to change patient response to illness in a positive manner. The expected outcome in the Nursing Process Balance model is the restoration of balance, or prevention of imbalance. The outcomes are measured in terms of physiological, psychological, physical, social, emotional, developmental, or spiritual behaviors that could be observed, described by the patient or others, and measured using standard instruments or equipment. For example, the expected outcome in a patient who is febrile is the reduction of body temperature back to normal. Using nursing interventions such as cooling measures, adjusting room temperature, and reducing the amount of clothing, can help bring body temperature back to normal, a state of balance. Collaborative nursing measures can also be employed along with primary nursing interventions such as administering anti-pyretic medications as ordered by the physician, or using cooling blankets in some cases. Sometimes, resolving a problem to achieve a certain outcome may require more than one intervention. Time frames should also be identified along with expected outcomes so that progress of the patient can be measured at certain points in time.

Nursing interventions are those actions of the nurse, whether direct or indirect that are performed based on clinical judgment directed towards meeting the desired outcomes. Nursing actions may be determined by the standards and protocols of the particular institution where he or she practices. These standards and protocols are intended to provide safe and therapeutic outcomes for the patients in that facility. However, these still require the independent clinical and professional judgment of the nurse. Interventions are aimed at the various clients that the nurse serves: individual patients, families, and community. Nursing interventions are also performed with rationales based on scientific principles. Evidence-based practice is the hallmark of professional nursing.

It is important to prioritize nursing interventions according to the order of the patient's most important needs. The Behavior Pyramid will give the nurse a guide to determine the most important needs at the time of interaction. Physiologic needs have to be satisfied first in order to meet the basic requirements of survival: air or oxygen, water or fluids, food or nutrition. Safety needs also have to be satisfied as part of survival. Once the physiologic needs are met, then psychological needs take precedence. Based on assessment data obtained, the psychological needs most important to the patient could be determined. For example, a patient who expresses anxiety over a surgical procedure has a need for information and to feel safe that the outcome of the surgery will be positive. This problem is causing an emotional imbalance on the patient that may affect his/her sleep, blood pressure, muscle tension, and cardiac function. This takes priority for nursing interventions over other needs at the moment because of the importance of maintaining emotional balance of the patient. Other approaches to allying the anxiety of the patient can also be employed that will ultimately contribute to the restoration of balance. Physiologic indicators will also show the effect of the nursing interventions such as lowering of blood pressure, heart rate, and relaxation of muscles.

Evaluation: Was balance achieved?

Evaluation is the process of determining whether a particular nursing intervention or set of interventions produced the desired outcome as determined through the nurse's clinical judgment. It is a continuous process in which the desired outcomes are used as the standard to determine if the nursing actions produced a change in behavior that is desirable in terms of bringing the patient to a state of equilibrium or balance. Nurses need to use their critical thinking process and their knowledge of scientific evidence to evaluate patient progress. Physiologic and psychosocial indicators have to be utilized in determining the efficacy of a particular intervention. For example, a patient who has a problem with blood sugar control needs to be evaluated using other criteria. The patient's compliance with the appropriate dietary guidelines should be evaluated. Additionally, other measures should be evaluated, such as the patient's exercise routine, attitude about his/her disease, family support, and access to resources. Blood sugar measurements should be correlated with these activities so that data generated will assist in more accurate evaluation.

The evaluation process requires that the nurse should ask some critical questions regarding the patient's progress: Has the patient's condition improved and to what extent? What are the indicators of this improvement? What are the patient's attitude and cultural beliefs about his illness that affect his/her compliance? Are there any barriers to the patient's ability to follow the appropriate regimen? Is the patient ready to accept changes in his/her lifestyle—if not, why not? A holistic approach, a basic approach to nursing care, should always be used to obtain a more comprehensive and individualized picture of the patient's condition. Because nursing is grounded on principles from different physical, psychological and social sciences, the nurse should be able to utilize this wide background to approach the patient's problems intelligently and scientifically.

The Nursing Process Balance model utilizes physiologic and psychosocial indicators in the evaluation process. Indicators are the measures of evidences that are needed to determine the outcome of interventions. Behavior is measured in terms of physiological, physical, and psychological changes that are verifiable through balance-seeking behaviors. The complexity of human behavior can only be appreciated by looking at the underlying systems within which human beings operate. Manifestations of balance seeking can be observed, described and measured as part of the evaluation process. The ultimate question that needs to be answered in evaluation is: was balance achieved by the client?

A comparison table between the steps of the traditional nursing process versus the Nursing Process Balance Model incorporating balance concepts is presented in Table 8.1.

KEY CONCEPTS

1. A Nursing Process Balance Model is proposed, using the concept of balance and nursing process as the basic frameworks for professional nursing practice. The steps of the traditional nursing process commonly used in nursing practice today are: assessment, nursing diagnosis identification, planning, implementation, and evaluation.

2. The first step in the nursing process is assessment where data are gathered about the patient's health status to establish a data base from primary and secondary sources. Cultural components and health behavior patterns are important aspects of assessment.

3. Nursing diagnosis is a clinical judgment about the response of the client (individual, family, or community) to actual and potential problems. The client's response is based on the analysis and interpretation of data gathered, clustered and prioritized to determine the patient's immediate and long-term problems and needs.

4. Planning involves the components of goal-setting, establishing priorities and selection of evidence-based appropriate interventions to meet desired patient outcomes. Goals determine the end-point of patient-care when met. Goals and expected outcomes have to be patient-centered, time-limited, observable, measurable, and realistic. Priority-setting is the step that involves ranking nursing diagnoses in their order of importance to the survival and well-being of the patient. Nursing interventions are then selected according to the problems identified.

5. Implementation of nursing interventions is the phase where actual performance of the selected nursing interventions are done based in clinical judgment, knowledge base, and skills of the nurse within their scope of practice. These actions are either directly or indirectly provided.

6. Evaluation is the fifth phase of the nursing but also a continuing process of determining whether the interventions provided produced the desired outcomes consistent with patient care goals.

7. While there are similarities with traditional nursing process, there are important differences with the Nursing Process Balance Model. A nursing process balance model incorporating the nursing process and the concept of balance is a framework for identifying the patient's state of balance or imbalance as a response to a problem or problems. It utilizes the same steps of the traditional nursing process but approaches problems using the balance/imbalance concepts. The proposed Nursing Process Balance model is designed to assist clients in moving back to a state of balance or equilibrium through the nursing process.

8. Assessment in the Nursing Process Balance model uses physiologic and psychosocial indicators, both quantitative and qualitative, as part of the data base. Cultural components are considered essential in obtaining data to provide a deeper understanding of the client's health care beliefs, attitudes and practices.

9. Nursing diagnosis is a statement of the specific imbalance identified during data assessment. This reflects the clinical judgment of the nurse based on critical thinking and problem solving by virtue of knowledge and skills from professional education and training.

10. Planning, goal-setting, and selection of nursing interventions are based on the imbalances identified as nursing diagnosis. Bringing the client back to a state of

balance and equilibrium, equivalent to a state of health and normalcy within the Zone of Equilibrium is always the goal of planning and care interventions.

11. Evaluation involves using the physiologic and psychosocial indicators that were used in assessment to identify the effects on patient outcomes—whether balance was reestablished and what needs to be done if the goals are not achieved.

CHAPTER 8: THE NURSING PROCESS BALANCE MODEL

REFERENCES

1. Daniels, R. 2004. *Nursing Fundamentals: Caring and Clinical Decision Making* (2nd ed.) New York. Delmar Thomson Learning.
2. Potter, P.A. and Perry, A.G. 2005. *Fundamentals of Nursing* (6th ed.) St. Louis, Missouri. Mosby.
3. NANDA International. 2005. *NANDA Nursing Diagnoses: Definitions and Classifications*, 2005-2006. Philadelphia.
4. Mosby Elsevier.2006. *Mosby's Dictionary of Medicine, Nursing & Health Professions* (7th ed.). St. Louis, Missouri. Mosby.
5. Carpenito-Moyet, L.J. 2008. *Nursing Diagnosis: Application to Clinical practice* (12th ed.). Philadelphia, PA. Lippincott Williams & Wilkins.
6. Alfaro-LeFebre, R. 1998. *Applying Nursing Diagnosis and Nursing Process: a Step-by-Step Guide* (4th ed.) Philadelphia, PA. Lippincott Williams and Wilkins.
7. Gordon, M. 1994. *Nursing Diagnosis: Process and Application* (3rd ed.) St. Louis. Mosby.
8. Dochterman, J.M. & Bulecheck, G.M. 2004. *Nursing Interventions Classification (NIC)* (4th ed.) St. Louis. Mosby.
9. Spector, R.E. 2004. *Cultural Diversity in Health and Illness* (7th ed.) Upper Saddle River, New Jersey. Pearson Prentice Hall.
10. Potter, P.A. & Perry, A.G. 2007. *Basic Nursing: Essentials for Practice* (6thed.) St. Louis, Missouri. Mosby.

TABLE 8.1 COMPARISON TABLE

STEPS IN THE TRADITIONAL NURSING PROCESS versus
THE NURSING PROCESS BALANCEMODEL

TRADITIONAL NURSING PROCESS	NURSING PROCESS BALANCE MODEL

1. ASSESSMENT DATA—primary and secondary sources
 	
a. Objective data
  • Physical assessment
  • Laboratory results
  • Diagnostic Procedures
b. Subjective data
  • Patient or client
  • Others—family, significant others, health care personnel
  • Relevant cultural data
	1. ASSESSMENT DATA: PHYSIOLOGIC, PSYCHO-SOCIAL INDICATORS—primary and secondary sources
	
	(Evidences of imbalance)
	
	a. Physiologic indicators from systems assessment (neurologic, respiratory, cardiovascular, endocrine, genito-urinary, digestive, musculo-skeletal,etc.)
	  • Physical assessment
	  • Laboratory results
	  • Diagnostic procedures
	b. Psychosocial indicators
	  • Subjective data
	  • Emotional behavior
	  • Spirituality
	  • Cultural data
	  • Knowledge level
	  • Maturational level

2. NURSING DIAGNOSIS (A clinical judgment about the client's responses to actual and potential health problems)
 	
  • NANDA diagnoses
    Actual nursing diagnosis
    Risk nursing diagnosis
    Wellness nursing diagnosis
	2. NURSING DIAGNOSIS (A statement of an imbalance in the physiologic, physical and psychosocial systems that can be changed through balance-seeking behaviors).
	
	  • Actual imbalance
	  • Potential or risk for imbalance
	  • Restoration of balance

3. PLANNING, GOAL-SETTING, INTERVENTIONS	3. PLANNING, GOAL-SETTING AND INTERVENTIONS
<ul><li>Outcomes-oriented</li><li>Goal-setting and priority-setting</li><li>Selecting interventions</li></ul>	<ul><li>Balance-oriented: restoration, maintenance of balance and prevention of imbalances</li><li>Outcomes directed towards balance in all aspects.</li><li>Interventions support balance-seeking behaviors.</li></ul>
4. IMPLEMENTATION (performance of nursing interventions to achieve goals and positive outcomes)	4. IMPLEMENTATION (performance of nursing interventions aimed at restoring, maintaining, supporting balance, and preventing imbalance).
<ul><li>Direct patient care</li><li>Indirect patient care</li><li>Collaborative care</li></ul>	<ul><li>Direct patient care</li><li>Direct patient care</li><li>Collaborative care</li></ul>
5. EVALUATION (ongoing process to determine if nursing interventions were effective in meeting goals and desired outcomes)	5. EVALUATION (ongoing process to determine if nursing interventions resulted in change in patient behavior and balance restored)
<ul><li>Reassessment and more data collection.</li><li>Re-set new goals to achieve desired outcomes.</li></ul>	<ul><li>Reassessment of balance state using more data from physiologic and psychosocial indicators.</li><li>Res-set new goals to achieve optimum state of balance within the zone of equilibrium.</li></ul>

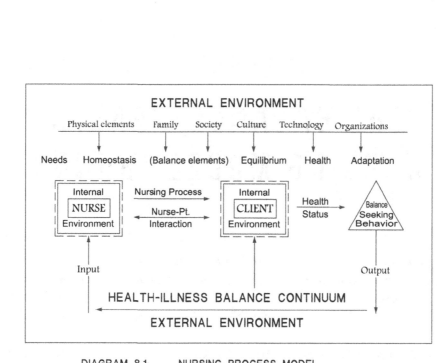

DIAGRAM 8.1:   NURSING PROCESS MODEL

Chapter 9

THE BALANCE-HEALTH NURSING MODEL (BHNM)

"Nursing is the protection, promotion, and optimization of health and abilities, prevention of illness and injury, alleviation of suffering through diagnosis and treatment of human response, and advocacy in the care of individuals, families, communities, and populations."
—American Nurses Association

Nursing is a discipline that is both an art and a science. The art is in delivering professional care in a compassionate, caring, and competent manner that respects the dignity of human beings. It is manifested in a manner that conveys a sincere attitude for the welfare of the client, consideration for the client's personal beliefs, empathy for their feelings, and a non-judgmental attitude. The ways that the nurse can demonstrate a caring attitude is as individual as the client and the nurse. The science of nursing has evolved over time. It is based on a body of knowledge that utilizes scientific evidence, research, new technology and discoveries, and knowledge obtained from other scientific fields. The development and testing of theories have contributed to this expanding body of knowledge and will continue to do so as long as nursing advances its growth as a profession.

As a discipline, nursing has taken a different path from that of the medical profession. Although medicine and nursing professionals have historically practiced side by side, nursing began to develop its own unique field of practice that can be distinguished from that of medicine. However, the public image of the nurse being subservient to the physician still lingers in today's real world. Nursing leaders have undertaken the goal of defining and expanding that body of knowledge that is unique to the profession through continued research and theory development. Professional practice has undergone major changes: clinical skills and competencies are enhanced through rigorous training; autonomy of practice safeguarded by state and federal regulations; client safety taking top priority thereby enhancing clinical practice; and participation in community and policy-making activities. All these have helped define the boundaries of modern nursing practice. The nursing profession is now enjoying the fruits of the labors of its leaders in its history through a greater sense of respect and acknowledgment of nurses' role in the health of the community and society.

THE METAPARADIGM OF NURSING: PERSON, HEALTH, ENVIRONMENT, AND NURSING

Knowledge in a particular discipline can be arranged in a hierarchical fashion. This can range from the abstract to concrete. Nursing has the body of knowledge that ranges from abstract to concrete. Nursing theories formulated by various theorists in the field have often based their models and constructs on abstract concepts. As nursing practice developed, it has increasingly used concrete evidence obtained from scientific researches and proven technology. It is replacing much of old practices born out of tradition and routine ways of doing things to the more solid evidence-based practice. Nursing is replete with traditions and practices that had been carried on through generations of nurses practicing their profession in whatever setting—hospitals, clinics, community centers, homes of clients, etc. But nursing practice has evolved over time as new knowledge, technology, and socio-cultural dynamics change. Like any other processes on this planet, nursing is also an evolving profession. A more well-defined science and practice of nursing is emerging.

There is another component of nursing practice that may have lost some of its emphasis due to the focus on research and hard scientific evidence. The humanistic element that separates nursing from other disciplines was losing ground as focus changed into healing the pathology, like the field of medicine, and less on the human being as more than the physical self. The perspective of nursing as an art was assuming less importance in the view of nursing as a science. This concern was not lost on early theorists who proposed a more holistic and caring approach. Well-known nursing theorists such as Watson, Neuman, Leininger, Rogers, and Newman suggested a new direction of caring for the whole person dynamically influenced by forces both within and outside of the individual. Foremost in the focus on caring is a theory by Jean Watson in the 1080's.[4,6] She developed the **Theory of Human Caring** and made the art and science of caring centrals concept in nursing. This places caring in the heart of nursing and the most central and unifying focus of nursing practice.[7] She was essentially an advocate for the humanization and holistic approach in nursing. The art of nursing is regaining its place in a rapidly changing world of high technology and scientific advances.

A discipline such as nursing has a unique perspective or manner with which it deals with phenomena within its boundary. For instance, medicine deals with pathology and treatment of diseases; psychology deals with human behavior and the psyche; sociology deals with people's social behavior; biology deals with the study of living organisms. Nursing is an interdisciplinary field which draws much of its philosophical foundations and practices from other fields. Nursing views all aspects of human beings from the broad context of environment, both internal and external, and beyond the immediate boundaries of daily experiences. The spiritual and existential aspects of the person's humanity affect behavior, health and well-being, and are integral parts of the culture that nurture each person. A particular view shared by a group of theorists within the discipline of nursing is called **a paradigm.** A more abstract view that serves to unify all points of views and perspectives within the discipline is called **metaparadigm.** The concepts within the metaparadigm define the limits and boundaries of the discipline.

The metaparadigm of nursing are: **person, environment, health**, and **nursing.**[2,4,6] All of these concepts intersect with the concept of balance. Balance serves as the foundation of these concepts. Survival is the impetus that gives rise to the forces of balance and its related elements. Without this drive for life itself, no living being can survive and life on earth as we know it would not exist. Knowledge, science, technology, culture and everything else will not amount to anything without first considering the forces of survival. Behavior unlocks the energy within each balance element and gives rise to survival mechanisms both inside the person's body and with the outside environment. Let us consider each of the four metaparadigm of nursing using the framework of the balance concept in selected nursing theories previously discussed.

Person

Nursing theorists base their assumptions on the metaparadigm of nursing that includes their concept of the person. In Roger's Theory of the Unitary Human Being, person is an **open system** in a continuous interaction with the environment, another open system. The human being is unitary, meaning that this entity is an irreducible, indivisible and multi-dimensional energy field that exists as a unified whole, whose sum is greater than its parts. Sister Callista Roy's Theory of Adaptation views humans as **adaptive systems** functioning as a whole. Human systems are not just individual human beings but also include systems that they created—families, organizations, communities, and society as a whole. Human systems have the capacity to adjust to and affected by the **environment** in the same manner as it affects the environment. Betty Neuman also utilizes the concept of **systems** and views the person as a system with multiple dimensions composed of physiological, psychological, socio-cultural, developmental, and spiritual factors. It is also considered an open system in dynamic interaction with the environment. Madeleine Leininger's Culture Care Theory considers **culture** as the values of individuals shared and learned with a particular group and transmitted from generation to generation. Culture influences a person's worldview and gives meanings to their perception of the world around them. Human interpretations, attitudes and beliefs, and social interactions reflect the influence of culture on their behavior.

The concept of "person" therefore has many interpretations, depending on the individual theorist's perspective. The balance framework defines person as a composite of multidimensional factors that affect behavior in response to internal and external stimuli. It is a living being, a product of the balancing forces of homeostasis, adaptation, equilibrium, needs and health. As a thinking, intelligent being, behavior is dictated by the expediencies confronting the individual, whether immediate or long-term, and makes choices influenced by individual needs. This presupposes that the individual is affected by internal and external forces of the environment and interacts with it constantly to ensure physical survival at the primal level, and psychosocial well-being at the higher levels. It also assumes that behavioral manifestations are reflections of the processing of inputs from within and without the physical being that operates as an open system. Evolutionary adaptations enabled it to adjust to the changing environment, including those that are beyond his conscious control. Internal physiologic needs were driven by automatic, innate processes that did not require conscious thought—such as the balancing forces of homeostasis and equilibrium. Balance-seeking behaviors are driven by internal and external factors, but all geared towards achieving balance and equilibrium, health and well-being, and ultimately, survival.

Other factors within the person include inherited characteristics and traits, personality, developmental stage, psychosocial factors, and spiritual beliefs that influence their ability to maintain mental balance and stability. The **Behavior Pyramid** based on Abraham Maslow's Hierarchy of Needs, identifies the particular realm of behavior associated with each level of need which ranges from the most basic physiologic to the highest level, the Self-fulfillment level. At the most basic level are those automatic and reflexive behaviors associated with the survival instinct. This instinct is the most primeval among humans. The rest of human behavior stems from this most basic instinct—life preservation. The combination of these complex factors and characteristics define what is called a **person.**

Environment

A dominant theme in many nursing theories is the role of the environment on human behavior and its effects on health. This concept of the environment as affecting people's health was first highlighted by Florence Nightingale. However, she had a limited view of environment compared to the broader perspective of later theorists. In her original writings, environment refers to those external elements that affect the sick and healthy individuals. This perhaps was owing to the limited scope of knowledge during her time, influenced by her direct experiences with the ravages of war on soldiers and the lack of sanitation in hospitals where she took care of ordinary citizens. This is still relevant in today's society where hazardous environmental conditions are matters of public health and safety.

A broader approach to the concept of environment was adopted by later scholars, namely Martha Rogers, Sister Callista Roy, Betty Neuman, Margaret Newman, and Madeleine Leininger. However, their definition of environment still differs from each other and the role it plays in behavior and health of human beings. Martha Rogers defines environment as an "energy field" identifiable by a pattern that is infinite, unpredictable, and characterized by diversity.[4] Environmental and human fields are integral with one another, suggesting a dynamic relationship. To Sister Callista Roy, environment consists of those stimuli that affect the person categorized as focal, contextual, and residual. The changing environment stimulates the person to make adaptive responses. Persons are adaptive systems that include internal and external factors. Betty Neuman believed in the reciprocal relationship between the person and the environment within a client system. Environment is defined as those internal and external factors that affect or interact with the person or client.[4] Stressors are factors in the environment that also interact and affect the person and could potentially destabilize the system. Margaret Newman's view of the environment, although not explicitly defined, is that level of consciousness beyond the consciousness of the individual. The assumption was based on the idea that all matters in the environment or universe possess consciousness but at different levels. Leininger's Cultural Care theory suggests culture as the context that gives meaning to people's experiences, expressions, interpretations, and social interactions. It could be inferred that culture is part of the individual's totality of experiences and reflect their worldview.

From the balance perspective, environment represents all those internal and external stimuli that influence or determine a person's behavior. The internal environment is composed of those physiologic and physical characteristics that function to maintain internal balance. These human characteristics include the brain, the command center of the body, biologically endowed and developed to the degree no other animal species possess. It controls both the response to outside stimuli as well as the regulation of the body's internal mechanisms to support basic life functions. Using the system theory, the person is viewed as an open system that is able to receive input via its anatomical and physiological capabilities, process this input or bits of information, and respond through behaviors that are observable, measurable and describable. Inputs come from both inside and outside the body.

The external environment consists not only of the physical elements, but also other people, such as family and community. The culture of the group where an individual belongs is part of the environmental context referred to by Leininger. The human being has physical and psychological boundaries that are permeable to stimuli from the external environment. There is a dynamic relationship between the person and the environment which is always in a state of flux. The individual is able to survive and thrive due to its ability to adapt to these changes physically and psychologically. Stressors are those factors in the environment that impinge and affect the person negatively through the mobilization of a generalized systemic response. To preserve balance and well-being, individuals use adaptive mechanisms to offset the negative effects of stressors. Some of these stressors are culturally determined, such as family relationships, jobs, role expectations, and cultural incongruence.

Health

The goal of nursing care is health. The problem with defining health, as we have found earlier in the book, is that there is no single definition that fits it in all instances. Although the World Health Organization has a definition that has been used as a frame of reference in many health care disciplines, it is still felt that it does not adequately capture the real essence of this term. Health is defined in many ways by the client and this is constantly changing. Each individual defines health differently. One's physical health status may be different from one's emotional health status. Or what one culture defines as healthy may not necessarily be true in another culture. Views of health can vary among different age groups, gender, race, and culture.[8] Health has been generally viewed as a continuum opposite with illness.

Nursing's overall concern is health. But most often, nursing encounters are when the client is ill and needs interventions or treatments to get them back to health. This concept was made quite clear when Florence Nightingale and her band of nurses during the Crimean War took care of soldiers to nurse them back to health. Nurses therefore provide care to clients throughout the health-illness continuum. While the emphasis on clients who are in a state of good health is maintenance and health promotion, and prevention of illness or disease, the emphasis on the illness side is returning the client back to a state of health. Failure to return the client back to health means increasing severity of the illness, and could lead to death. Illness poses a threat to the life of the client and his continued survival. Nursing is concerned with the whole spectrum of health and illness of the client. Doing this requires consideration of all aspects of the individual: physical, psychological, emotional, cultural, and spiritual. It also requires knowing the environmental factors that affect the person and how he or she responds to them.

To understand health and illness, models have been developed to obtain greater insight into the relationship between these concepts and the client's view of health, their healthcare attitudes and beliefs, their determinants of health, as well as their health behaviors. There are several nursing models developed by various nurses:[2,6] The **Health Belief Model** by Rosenstoch, Becker and Maiman (1975), **Health Promotion Model (HPM)** by Nola Pender (1982, 1996), **Basic Human Needs Model** by Abraham Maslow (discussed elsewhere in the book), **Holistic Health Models.** The Health Belief Model is based on the premise that there is a relationship between a person's beliefs and behaviors. This model helps nurses understand the factors influencing clients' beliefs, attitudes, perceptions and behaviors in order to plan the most effective way of promoting health for the client. Nola Pender's Health Promotion Model aims to promote health by considering all the variables affecting the client's health. The desired outcome of this model is health-promoting behavior achieved through modifying the variables that negatively impact health. The Basic Human Needs Model by Abraham Maslow has provided an important understanding of human behavior in terms of how human needs are met. These needs are arranged in a hierarchy, starting with the most basic physiologic need to the highest level, self-actualization. Holistic Models considers the important dimensions of the clients, including spiritual and emotional well-being. The client is in control of their health behaviors, involved in their healing process, and assumes self-responsibility to maintain their health.

Health is an important element in the balance concept because it is what keeps the physical, emotional, and psychosocial well-being of the client in a state of balance. An optimal state of health is the desired outcome of nursing process. Most of the time, the nurse provides care at the opposite end of the continuum, when the clients get sick. The nurse's role in the balance equation is most evident when involved in life and death situations where the actions, critical thinking, and clinical expertise of the nurse can save the client's life. This critical condition is a state of extreme imbalance when disease or illness progresses. When the human being's physical and physiologic state are placed at risk through severe illness or life-threatening situations, the nursing actions to bring the client back to a state of stability requires close monitoring of life indicators such as vital signs.

Nursing

Nursing's metaparadigm has a broader scope than many other disciplines. It deals with the interaction between the nurse and the client and is concerned with all human aspects. It has a holistic approach that makes nursing a unique discipline. However, each nursing theory presents a different view of these metaparadigm concepts.[6]Martha Rogers views nursing's focus as people and their environments. She identified the purpose of nursing as the promotion of health and well-being of all people. It is both an art and a science, a view that has been adopted and accepted by most nursing leaders. The art of nursing uses science in various ways to assist in the life processes of humans. It promotes and strengthens human and environmental fields to achieve maximum potential.[4] Jean Watson focuses more on the art of caring, a concept she had made as central to nursing. It stems from her philosophy and belief in humanistic and altruistic values applied to the practice of nursing.

Sister Callista Roy's view of nursing is somewhat similar to that of Rogers in that Roy broadly defines nursing as a health care profession that focuses on human life processes and patterns and emphasizes promotion of health for individuals, families, groups and society as a whole. She emphasizes enhancing and expanding the person's adaptive abilities and promoting health. Enhancing the person's ability to interact positively with the environment promotes adaptation in each of the four adaptive modes. Betty Neuman believes in caring for the client as a whole person. This means being concerned with all the variables affecting the person and the individual's response to stressors in the environment. These stressors are interpersonal, intrapersonal, or extrapersonal as a result of people's dynamic interaction with the environment, seen as an open system. The nurse functions in three levels of prevention—primary, secondary, and tertiary, in order to reduce the effects of stressors and achieve a state of wellness, meaning system needs are being met.

THE BALANCE HEALTH NURSING MODEL (BHNM) AND MAJOR ASSUMPTIONS

Integrating the balance concepts into the practice of nursing appears logical and theory-based. Understanding the universality of balance, its core elements, the concepts of environment (internal and external), human behavior, culture and health, all point to the need for a unified nursing model. The centrality of balance in health, well-being, and survival is now better understood. The major concepts that are the foundations of the domain of nursing—person, health, environment and nursing—are all within the framework of balance. Using balance as the concept that closely interweaves and knits the fabric of nursing together gives a more integrated approach to nursing practice. Common elements of a balance nursing model can be drawn from various selected theories. Elements and concepts found in these selected nursing theories such as health, illness, wellness, environment, open systems, behavior, adaptation, homeostasis, needs, equilibrium, harmony, stability, etc. are all related to balance. Based on these theoretical and evidence-based foundations, an integrated model of health, balance, and nursing is proposed called the **BALANCE HEALTH NURSING MODEL** (DIAGRAM 9.1).

The **Balance Health Nursing Model (BHNM)** incorporates the Nursing Process Model and the Behavior Pyramid within the Health-illness Balance continuum as the totality of the health care environment within which nursing practices as a member of the health care professions. It is based on the following major assumptions encompassing the metaparadigm of nursing: person, environment, health, and nursing:

Person

A person is a biological and spiritual being endowed with intellectual, creative, and adaptive capacities superior to any other species on earth. The human being shares some common elements with the external environment, affected by it, and interacts dynamically with it.

It naturally possesses the anatomic and physiological structures and systems to receive stimuli from the environment, processes these internally, and manifests its response through behavior. The instinct for **survival** has enabled it to continue its existence on the planet via mechanisms and behaviors that are innate, reflexive or automatic, adaptive, physiologic, and need-satisfying. **Balance** and its core elements that exist internally and externally serve as the basic structures of survival. These elements are **equilibrium, homeostasis, adaptation, needs and health**. **Behavior** serves as the switch that turns on these elements from the beginning of its life. Behavior is a movement driven by an energy source from the internal and external environment performed both internally and externally in response to physiological, physical, psychological, and sociological stimuli. These behaviors tend to seek balance to maintain **stability** and **equilibrium** in their existence.

The human being is also a social animal, stemming from its most primal origin of mother-child and family relationships characteristic of mammals. **Evolutionary processes**, aided primarily by a superior brain, have evolved human beings physically, socially, and psychologically into the modern person. The humans we know today is a highly sophisticated, social, dynamic, and intelligent being within a variety of cultures and social organizations that it developed over time. It has found new aspirations to satisfy not just basic physiologic needs but also higher psychosocial needs to find self-fulfillment. **Balance-seeking** also found expressions in spirituality, harmony, creativity, equality, and well-being. Inability to find balance results in an **imbalance**—manifested in illness and disease. Grave imbalances can lead to death. Imbalances threaten the health, well-being, and survival of human beings.

Another characteristic of human beings as a living, biologic entity is its **adaptive** capacity. This ability to adjust and undergo changes physically and psychologically enabled it to survive environmental, social, and psychological elements over time since the beginning of its existence. Adaptive mechanisms have been at work since time immemorial. The physical adaptive changes were part of the evolutionary process apparently intended by nature to maintain human survival on the planet. Psychological adaptive mechanisms are processes that persons use to deal with stressors from the environment. The goal of both physical and psychological adaptive mechanisms is survival.

Health

The complexity of the concept of health and the difficulty of giving it one precise definition has been discussed. The Balance Health Nursing Model presents its own view about health within the context of **human survival**. Human beings survive through the preservation of its life processes. Life is supported by basic necessities such as air, food, water and shelter. These are called basic needs in **Maslow's Hierarchy of Needs** discussed elsewhere in the book and compose the physiologic elements necessary to maintain life at the cellular level. Without these elements to feed and nourish the cells, the physical body will die. In the hierarchy of needs, these are the things that come first before any other priorities. Although not immediately needed for survival, sex is included in this category because the human race will not continue to survive without propagating itself through sexual activity.

Health has been viewed as a **continuum** with illness. Theorists use this perspective as a major assumption. Betty Neuman views health as a continuum of wellness to illness that is dynamic in nature and subject to change.[4,5] Because of this dynamic nature, a client's state of either wellness or illness can change and at any given point in time. Unmet system needs create a decreased state of wellness. Health is a major concept in Margaret Newman's Theory of Expanding Consciousness. Health is viewed as a merging of the concepts of disease and nondisease to create a larger whole. Health is a pattern of the whole, encompassing the consciousness of the person and the environment. This is consistent with the holistic view of health encompassing the totality of the human being in dynamic interaction with the environment.

The **Balance Health Nursing Model** proposes that health is a **range of states** between health and illness as defined by the individual, placing the concept of health within the **health-illness continuum**. Each person defines their state of health from their own perspective, that could be validated by observations, measurements, and self-report of the individual. There has to be a certain level of congruence between objective measures with how the patient describes his or her condition and the objective results of measurement tools. The only way this can be determined is through assessment and evaluations of **behavioral manifestations**. With modern techniques and methods of assessing **health status** of individuals, their definition of health can be reliably validated. A state of **optimum health** or well-being is a state of total balance of the individual in all aspects of its life—physical, psychological, emotional, and spiritual. This is the zone of equilibrium within the health-illness continuum. Illness is a state of imbalance, where the individual's state of health and well-being are compromised. Continued imbalance will lead to death without definitive interventions.

An imbalanced health can be restored, and optimum health can be maintained and achieved through **balance-seeking behaviors**. Individuals must engage in balance-seeking behaviors, or support balance processes to reach a level of health. Failure by individuals to support its balance-seeking functions will result in ill-health and imbalance. There has to be a conscious effort of the individual to find the level of health that is compatible with his or her definition of well-being. An unmet need must be met—whether it is physical, physiologic, psychological, emotional, and intellectual to reach their self-defined level of self-fulfillment. To do this, the individual must use certain adaptive mechanism to enable them to adapt or adjust to constant changes within their internal and external environments. This stems from the innate capacity of human beings for adaptation, a characteristic that serves them well in the course of their constant struggle for survival, from the harshness of the savannahs in primitive societies to the boardrooms of the modern world.

Modern societies have developed health care systems to care for individuals when they are ill—from diseases, infections, malfunctions, traumas, or mental illness. These schools of thought, whether from the western medicine perspective, or the eastern medicine and alternative medicine perspective, are all intended to heal individuals from these states of imbalance and preserve life. Ancient practices of medicine dealt with crude methods of healing. Nursing dealt with environmental issues but also geared towards restoring health and promoting healing in patients. Modern health care as we know it, is still constantly evolving and will continue to evolve as new inventions and discoveries change the way health care is delivered. Nurses within these health care systems will continue to find ways to improve outcomes in the practice of the nursing profession.

Environment

The **environment** is the sum of all factors **internal and external** that surrounds, affects, influences, and interacts with all human beings. Internal environment refers to the physiologic elements inside the body that maintains internal **equilibrium** and **homeostasis**. It also refers to the body's internal mechanisms responsible for generating physiologic and psychological response. The human brain is largely responsible for determining the body's responses via its neurologic control systems. As much as the body responds to internal signals, it also responds to external signals from the environment. The human body is an open system that receives **input** or stimuli from the external environment, processes the information, and produces outputs in terms of behavior.

As an **open system**, the human being has parts that compose a whole that interacts with the environment. This is a holistic view of human beings. The various parts in an open system are organized and interrelated to produce a whole. The output is not simply the sum total of its independent parts but assumes a different quantity. The human behavioral output as a result of its dynamic interaction with the internal and external environments defines the individuality of human beings. Response to stimuli from the **internal environment** can be determined by one's physical state of health, inherited traits, personality, mental state, experiences, and other psychological factors. Different aspects of behavior reflect the influences of these internal factors.

The **external environment** is composed of physical environmental elements and all other factors outside of the person's body that affect or influence it in various ways. These include family, community, society, culture, organizations, and technological innovations that change people's lives. The external environment can be a major factor in health. It is also a source of stress and emotional imbalance. The negative effects of stress on the body was described by Selye as a physiologic response called the General Adaptation Syndrome (GAS).[2,6] This close interrelationship between the internal and external environments is made possible because of the permeability of human beings to receive **stimuli** from the outside as well as respond to it.

Nursing

The discipline of nursing has two components: the theoretical **body of knowledge** and nursing **practice.** The theory and practice must be congruent: theory and practice go hand in hand. Various nursing theorists define nursing according to their locus of interests. The earliest definition of nursing was by Florence Nightingale who described the role of nurses as having the responsibility to care for someone's health. Sister Callista Roy in her Adaptation Theory defines nursing as the science and practice that expands adaptive abilities and enhances person and environmental transformation.[3,4] Central to her definition is the concept of adaptation. The goal of nursing, according to Roy, is geared towards the promotion of adaptation for the clients (individuals and groups). Betty Neuman's Systems Model views nursing as a profession participating actively in all the variables affecting the individual's response to stressors.[4,5] The five variables that comprise the whole system of the client—physiological, psychological, sociocultural, developmental, and spiritual—affect the client's interaction with the environment. In Madeleine Leininger's Culture Care, nursing refers to a learned humanistic and scientific profession whose focus is on care that are culturally meaningful and beneficial to the client.[4] A more modern definition of nursing is that of the American Nurses Association which states: "Nursing is the protection, promotion, and optimization of health and abilities, prevention of illness and injury, alleviation of suffering through diagnosis and treatment of human response, and advocacy in the care of individuals, families, communities, and populations."[1]

These views suggest several major components of the essence of nursing: 1) it is concerned with **managing behavior,** 2) it is an **interpersonal relationship** between nurse and client, and 3) it involves a **process** to achieve its goals. The goal of nursing is to help clients achieve positive outcomes in their health and well-being through various roles. Professional responsibilities and roles of nurses include the following: caregiver, educator, advocate, communicator, leader, manager, and coordinator of care. These roles also carry corresponding ethical and legal obligations of the profession to their clients. These definitions suggest a common theme—that the nurse is concerned with influencing client behaviors, to change or modify outcomes towards the improvement of their condition or status. Nursing becomes involved in client care when there is a need for care that nurses provide. That point is where clients have developed a certain state of need—whether physiologic, psychological, or socio-cultural—that affects the client's health and well-being. Nurses' interaction with their clients start the moment there is an interpersonal contact. The point of contact is when the nurse assumes responsibility for the care of the client.

The ultimate goal of the nurse is to get the client into a state of health or wellness through actions or interventions utilizing the **nursing process.** The use of this process, utilizing critical thinking, is what distinguishes nursing from other disciplines such as medicine. It considers the individuality of the client, who is an active participant in the process. The ultimate outcome is a comprehensive, individualized approach to care.[2] The nursing process is inherent in the definition of the American Nurses Association as a process that utilizes methods to identify, diagnose, and treat **human responses** to health and illness. Response, as we know, refers to the behavior of the individual. In essence, nursing is involved in modifying client behavior to effect changes for the betterment of the client's health and well-being. These are desired outcomes of the nursing process and the overall goal of nursing. To put it simply, nursing is involved in modifying client behaviors that will bring positive outcomes.

The **nursing process** necessarily involves nurse-client interaction and brings forth the factors that are nurse-determined and client-determined. The client brings health care needs, expectations, attitudes, beliefs, cultural background, educational background, and other socio-psychological factors to the interaction. Similarly, the nurse also brings all these factors, as well as her/his educational preparation, knowledge and skills. The nursing process is a dynamic process of interpersonal exchange and communication between the nurse and the client. As in traditional nursing process, the model also involves five essential steps: **assessment**, **nursing diagnosis**, **planning**, **implementation**, and **evaluation**. The goal of the nursing process is to influence and change the behavior (human response) of clients to improve or maintain the client's level of health and well-being. Clients refer to individuals, family, and community which the nurse accepted responsibility for caring.

DEFINITIONS AND MAJOR CONCEPTS

The Balance Health Nursing Model (**BHNM**) proposes this definition of nursing: "*Nursing is the science and art of restoring, maintaining, and promoting balance, and preventing imbalance of the client through management and modification of behavior using the nursing process within the health-illness continuum*".

The following are the major concepts and definitions in the model:

Balance—Balance is the dynamic interplay of all forces that equalize each other within the internal and external environments of the person. It is the energy that serves as the foundation of those processes that enable human beings to survive. It is the essence of survival. Balance has five essential elements which interact synergistically with each other to form the core of survival: homeostasis, equilibrium, adaptation, needs and health. The balance concept is universally found in all aspects of life and fields of study: the physical sciences, social sciences, health professions, economics, architecture, engineering, arts, religion, culture, etc. Balance is the essential element in health and creates stability, harmony, and well-being.

Imbalance—Imbalance is a state of relative disequilibrium or instability and is the opposite concept of balance. It is a state where forces do not equalize each other. Continued imbalance places the health and well-being of individuals at risk.

Equilibrium—Equilibrium is a state where opposing or competing forces cancel each other out thereby producing a state of balance. It is an imaginary zone in the center of positive and negative elements that has the most harmony.

Adaptation—It is the process by which human beings and all living beings modify themselves over time to adjust to changing situations and environmental conditions. The goal of adaptation is continued survival.

Homeostasis—The state of dynamic equilibrium of the internal environmental of the body to maintain a state of stability by regulating its physiologic processes.

Needs—Something that is wanting or lacking in the individual, or deemed necessary by the individual, that has to be met. Unmet needs result in imbalance.

Survival—It is the innate impetus of all human beings to preserve life. All basic life processes are geared towards survival.

Behavior—An observable, measureable, and describable response to stimuli in the internal and external environments of a person. Behavioral responses are in three realms: physical, biological, and psychosocial. The ultimate goal of behavior is to find balance.

Behavior Pyramid—A hierarchy of behavior based on Maslow's Hierarchy of Needs that defines the various realms of behavior according to its level of importance to the survival and psychological well-being of a person. There are four realms of behavior from the most basic to the highest realm of behavior: 1) Reflexive or automatic realm, 2) Emotional and spiritual realm, 3) Intellectual and rational realm, 4) Self-fulfillment and balance. The development of these realms of behavior follow the order of human development in the evolutionary process.[11]

Reflexive behavior are those dictated by physiologic needs that are basic for immediate survival such as air, water, food, and safety. This behavior is affected by both internal and external factors that trigger a basic response. This is the first level of behavior that human beings have in common with other animals on the planet and the first to be developed in the process of man's evolution. The seat of this behavior lies in the brain stem—the earliest part of the brain to develop.

Emotional and Spiritual behaviors are those behaviors that stem from the nature of man as a social being. These are the needs for love, self-esteem, belongingness, friendship, acceptance, sexual drive, and spiritual relationship with a Supreme Being. The emotional behavior is governed by the limbic system in the brain that developed next in the evolutionary ladder.

Intellectual/rational behaviors are those behaviors that are the results of intellectual processes and rational thought, analysis of data, scientific approach, use of logic, and knowledge from known sources. The intellect, personality, the logical part of the brain, and the artistic brain are said to be housed in the cerebral cortex, the seat of all human consciousness.

Self-fulfillment and balance is the highest level achievable by any human being. This is the level where a person finds complete satisfaction and fulfillment beyond his basic physiologic needs. Higher psychosocial needs in the emotional, spiritual, and intellectual realms have been met and the person achieves a complete sense of fulfillment. This is the level where a person finds the most balance and equilibrium in life. However, self-fulfillment is defined only by the person himself or herself according to the standards that the person has determined.

Balance-seeking behaviors—are those set of behaviors whose goal is to find balance in the physiologic, physical, and psychological realms through adaptive mechanisms.

Adaptive mechanisms—are the physiologic, physical and psychological means which individuals utilize in order to adapt or adjust to stimuli from the internal and external environments to enable balance-seeking to find fulfillment of its goals.

Environments—are conditions or forces present both within (internal or intrinsic) and outside (external or extrinsic) the person's physical being that directly or indirectly affect the person's behavior.

Health—is the sum total of the person's response to internal and external stimuli that defines the person's state of balance derived from adaptive mechanisms. It is a measure of the person's state of balance along health-illness continuum.

Open system—is a system whose elements are in dynamic interaction with inputs and outputs. Human beings are open systems as well as a part of the larger system in a world filled with stimuli. The sources of stimuli come from within the internal environment of the person, as well as the external environment. Human beings have the capability to receive stimuli (input) and respond to it (output). A feedback mechanism allows for dynamic changes within the systems.

Nursing Process—an orderly logical process of identifying clients' degree of imbalance and implementing interventions to modify human responses to restore and maintain health, and prevent illness. This process has five essential steps: assessment, nursing diagnosis, planning, implementation, and evaluation. It requires nurse-patient interaction.

Nurse-patient interaction—a dynamic relationship between the nurse and the patient that involves communication, exchange of information, and backgrounds that both bring to the relationship. The nurse and the client both bring different perspectives, beliefs, attitudes, personality and behaviors to the situation. The nurse assumes the professional role in this interaction by virtue of his or her education, training, professional standards, and ethical-legal obligations.

A FRAMEWORK FOR PROFESSIONAL PRACTICE

The Balance Health Nursing Model (**BHNM**) as proposed is intended to provide a broader framework of professional nursing practice based on a universal concept: BALANCE. *The core concepts of this model are those that contribute to the ultimate goal of achieving the highest level of balance in the client utilizing the nursing process.* It is incorporated with the health-illness balance continuum to provide the broadest scope of nursing practice. The process starts when the nurse establishes a nurse-patient relationship, known as the nurse-patient interaction. The client could be an individual person, family, or community. As the "client" becomes more diverse, the factors that they bring into the nurse-patient interaction become more complex. The nurse is a human being first and affected by the same internal and external factors affecting the client. The client and the nurse both move within a health-illness continuum.

The desired outcomes of the nursing process are the **balance-seeking behaviors** of the client to meet needs within the Behavior Pyramid. In an open system, this is the output. To meet client's needs in the Behavior Pyramid, adaptive mechanisms are required in order to meet needs in each level successfully and maintain balance, whether in the physiological, or psychological realms. The nurse assists the client in meeting those needs through **modifying behaviors** that cause imbalance. For instance, a client in respiratory difficulty can be given oxygen as ordered by the physician and after assessment by the nurse. Respiratory difficulty is an imbalanced behavior observed in a client. To bring the client back to a state of balance requires modifying or changing this behavior through interventions such as reassuring the client, positioning, decreasing activity, and administering oxygen. Once the respiratory problem is decreased or corrected, the client goes back to a balanced state. An emotional imbalance can be addressed through adaptive mechanisms that utilize **coping mechanisms**. For instance, an anxious client becomes unstable, imbalanced. Through the actions of the nurse employing the client's adaptive coping mechanisms, such as providing information, using family and community resources, anxiety can be reduced and balanced can be restored.

How do you define positive outcomes behaviorally? Behavior can be assessed through observations, measurements and self-descriptions by the client. In utilizing the balance concept as a frame of reference, outcomes pertain to the state of balance of the individual client within the health-illness continuum. The closer the client gets to the zone of equilibrium, the more optimal his or her state of health. The nursing process is therefore geared towards achieving positive outcomes—bringing the client as close to a state of balance and equilibrium as possible through actions aimed at modifying client behaviors. For instance, an immobile client who is uncomfortable in a certain position and unable to sleep is feeling a state of imbalance. This can be changed by putting the client in a more comfortable position and instituting some comfort measures such as back rubs to relieve the area of discomfort. As a result, the client's discomfort is relieved and able to sleep eventually—a positive outcome from behavior modification (changing position). This outcome started with an assessment of the client's discomfort, making a diagnosis, carrying out interventions that involved some degree of planning, and evaluation of the effects of the intervention. Had the interventions been ineffective to make the client comfortable (a state of imbalance), then the client's status needs to be re-evaluated to change to a positive outcome.

The patient **open system** provides feedback to the nurse via the nursing process. This behavioral output becomes the input that the nurse uses to evaluate the effectiveness of planning and interventions employed. This provides the information the nurse needs to determine the client's health status and his/her place in the health-illness continuum. The client also interacts with the environment and obtains information/data from the external environment. The type of family support or community support obtained is his/her feedback from the external environment. The culture where the client belongs provides input as to the attitudes, beliefs, and cultural practices within the culture that support or negate the client behavior. This will help in determining the adaptive mechanisms that the client need to employ to find psychological balance.

The nurse and the patient/client both exist and function within a health-illness balance continuum where internal and external factors are always at play. The nurse brings her own skills, knowledge, cultural background, professional and life experiences, societal influences, family and community relationships, organizational factors, attitudes and beliefs, and health status to the situation. All these define the totality of her/his being in the same manner that these are the same factors that the client brings to the relationship and interaction. Both exist within a health-illness balance continuum that define their individual environments. However, the difference is that nurses have the ability to assess health status and modify or change a client's behavior to produce positive outcomes, directing them towards balance-seeking behaviors. The nurse-client relationship is a unique relationship in that the nurse has the dominant role of bringing about balance in the lives of the client owing to the practitioner's superior knowledge and skills in the nursing process. The nursing model recognizes the important role that nurses play in changing the lives of patients.

EMPERICAL EVIDENCES

The theoretical foundations of the concept of balance are well-recognized in the scientific community. In the diverse fields of science, the balance concept has been used since time immemorial. From Galileo, to Newton, to all those other famous scientists of long ago who discovered the nature of the earth and its principles have used the concept of balance. The ancients understood its meaning when they used instruments to measure their goods and precious stones. The primitive peoples around the world intuitively understood balance in their worship of nature and the earth's harmony with its spirit. Artists and artisans for centuries sensed balance through their artistry in their creations. The healers from ancient times understood the importance of treating illness, a state of imbalance, to get back to a state of health or balance. All the collective knowledge of human beings have the elements of balance imbedded in their DNA. Within the human body are stable, basic structures and processes that continue its work as long as it is alive. This is how human beings have been able to survive up to this time. The concept of open systems, although of recent vintage comparatively speaking, was important in greatly understanding the role of the environment, human behavior and the dynamic interactions between them. The evolutionary process in the history of human development continues as long as humans possess the capacity for adaptation. Theories will continue to be developed in the search for greater understanding of this living thing called human being. It is with confidence that the author proposes that a model of balance is a universal model that applies to nursing practice and health care.

The specific nursing theories that are used in developing this model are those of Florence Nightingale (environment), Betty Newman (System Model), Sister Callista Roy (Adaptation), Dorothy Johnson (Behavioral Systems), Madeleine Leininger (Cultural Care), and Jean

Watson (Caring). Additionally, theories from the sociological and physical sciences formed the basic ideas relevant to the balance concept. Principles from the fields of physics, chemistry, sociology, psychology, economics, ecology, and anthropology laid the ground works for developing the balance concepts. It is this multidisciplinary approach that has provided the critical understanding of the nature of balance. Most of all, it is the search for a greater meaning of the humanity of man that has driven this endeavor.

KEY CONCEPTS

1. The concepts in the metaparadigm of nursing—person, health, environment and nursing—are all concepts encompassed in the nursing process within the health-illness balance continuum. Balance serves as the frame of reference within which nursing provides care that preserves the survival, health, and wellbeing of the person through management and influencing changes in behavior within its environments.

2. Nursing scholars have varying views of the person, health, environment and the goals of nursing. Their theories and views have validity and are useful in the continued development of scientific thought in nursing. These were also explored and considered in the development of the Balance Health Nursing Model (BHNM).

3. Key concepts used in the Balance Health Nursing Model (**BHNM**) are: balance, imbalance, equilibrium, adaptation, homeostasis, needs, survival, behavior, Behavior Pyramid, balance-seeking behavior, internal and external environments, health, adaptive mechanisms, open system, nursing process, nurse-client interaction.

4. The BHNM is based on the core concepts of the nursing process within the health-illness balance continuum. Major assumptions center around the metaparadigm of nursing (person, environment, health and nursing), the nursing process, the behavior pyramid, health-illness, and the concept of balance/imbalance. This is what makes the BHNM different from other nursing models. With balance as its unifying framework, a more universal and comprehensive approach is presented.

5. The nurse-patient interaction using the nursing process defines the relationship between the patient/client and the nurse. This is where nursing applies its best practices through the steps of the nursing process—from the assessment of client health status, to identification of nursing diagnosis, planning, interventions and evaluation. Balance is used as a frame of reference in assessing health status and behavioral patterns. Caring interventions strengthen the nurse-patient relationship, reinforce balance, and bring positive outcomes.

6. The theoretical foundations of the BHNM are derived from scientific thoughts and theories developed over time—evidences of the relevance of the balance concept in many aspects of life and health.

CHAPTER 9: THE BALANCE HEALTH NURSING MODEL (BHNM)

REFERENCES

1. American Nurses Association. 2003. *Standards of Nursing Practice* (ed. 3). Washington, DC. The Association.
2. Potter, P. A. and Perry, A.G. 2005. *Fundamentals of Nursing* (6th ed.) St. Louis, Missouri. Mosby.
3. Roy, C. & Andrews, H. 1999. *The Roy Adaptation Model* (2nd ed.) Stamford, CT. Appleton & Lange.
4. Tomey, A.M. & Alligood, M.R. 2002. *Nursing Theorists and their Work* (5th ed.) St. Louis, Missouri. Mosby, Inc.
5. Freese, B. 2002. "Betty Neuman: Systems Model". in Tomey, A.M. & Alligood, M.R. 2002. *Nursing Theorists and their Work (5th ed.)* Norwalk, CT. Appleton-Century-Crofts.
6. Daniels, R., Grendell, R.N. & Wilkins, F.R. 2004. *Nursing Fundamentals* (2nd ed.) Clifton Park, New York. Delmar.
7. Neil, R.M. 2002. Jean Watson: Philosophy and Science of Caring". in Tomey, A.M. & Alligood, M.R. 2002. *Nursing Theorists and their Work (5th ed.)* Norwalk, CT. Appleton-Century-Crofts.
8. Pender, N.J. 1996. *Health Promotion and Nursing Practice* (3rd ed.). Stamford, CT. Appleton & Lange.
9. Lewis, S.L., Heitkemper, M.M. & Dirksen, S.R. 2007. *Medical-Surgical Nursing: Assessment and Management of Clinical Problems* (7th ed.) South Asia edition. St. Louis, Missouri. Mosby.
10. American Nurses Association: *Nursing's Social Policy Statement*. Washington, DC. The Association.
11. *Rayner, C. (cont. Ed.) 1980. Funk & Wagnalls Atlas of the Body.* New York. Rand McNally & Company.

DIAGRAM 9.1: THE BALANCE HEALTH NURSING MODEL (BHNM)

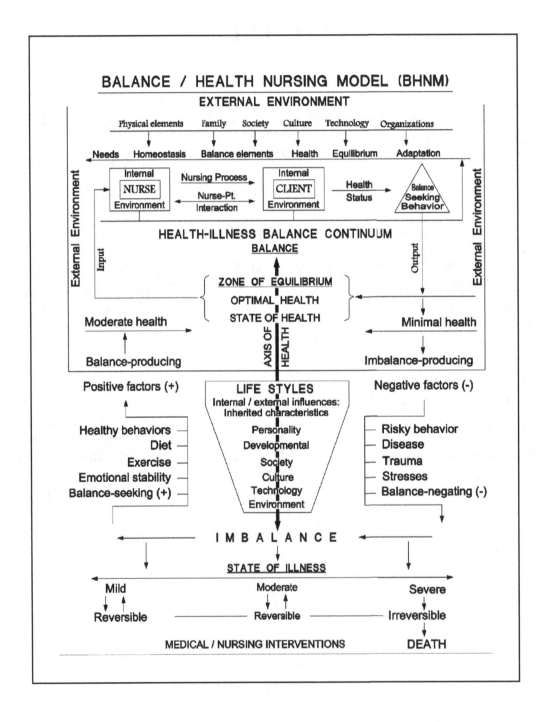

Chapter 10

BALANCE HEALTH ASSESSMENT TOOL AND APPLICATION

People are like stained-glass windows. They sparkle and shine when the sun is out, but when the darkness sets in their true beauty is revealed only if there is light from within.
~Elisabeth Kübler-Ross

PURPOSES OF TOOL

A health assessment tool based on the Balance Health Nursing Model was developed that can be used by professional nurses in applying the nursing process to provide care for their clients. It is a tool that can be used in obtaining a set of data about the client to determine health status which reflects the state of balance of the client. It was purposely designed with simplicity in mind in order for it to be a useful tool in data-gathering and not cumbersome work that sometimes accompanies data-gathering tools in some places. This tool will also be useful in the training and education of nursing students by providing them with a basic instrument to learn assessment skills. By going thru the process of obtaining data, it enhances the student's skills in interviewing, establishing rapport with patients, and identifying problems and potential problems. The best opportunity to use this tool is upon admission to a hospital or facility to obtain basic general information on the client and to organize a **data base.** A complete data base includes a thorough health history, physical assessment, and psychosocial assessment.[1] It then enables the health care practitioner to have enough data to establish a nursing diagnosis. These then become the basis for writing an individualized **nursing care plan** for each client.

Important considerations

Use of the Balance Health Assessment Tool entails some important considerations:

1. Balance assessment.

It is important to approach the Balance Health Assessment Tool from the perspective of balance assessment—that the health status of patients is determined by the degree of balance or imbalance present in the patient in all aspects of existence. This is the core concept upon which the Balance Health Nursing Model is based. The overall state of health of the patient depends on the degree that the person is able to establish a sense of well-being and balance. This does not just depend on physical health. It also depends on the degree the person is able to meet psychological, emotional, and spiritual needs. An optimum state of health and balance is the goal of human existence. In the Behavior Pyramid, this is the ultimate state where self-fulfillment is achieved.

2. Prioritization

By looking at the primary physiologic assessment data first—the **ABC** (airway, breathing, and circulation), the primacy of survival is established. These are vital physiologic functions that have to be present for the patient to survive. Establishing responsiveness to stimuli takes first priority by looking at the neurologic/cognitive function. Next is establishing patency of the airway by assessing the respiratory system. The circulatory function is then assessed by establishing presence of pulses and blood pressure. Secondary assessment includes other systems that are important but not immediately needed for survival. For the body to maintain a completely well-balanced entity, all the body organs and systems have to be in good working condition. Disorder of one system or organ can affect the entire body and throw the entire being in a state of imbalance.

3. Organization of data

Both quantitative and qualitative data should be included in the assessment to obtain a more complete assessment of the patient's health. Data obtained must be organized and **clustered** to form a data base. Before the nurses can make sense of these data, they must have the background knowledge in anatomy, physiology, sociology, psychology, the physical sciences and other related fields to correlate these information with patient health status. Clustering data enables the nurse to identify patterns of cues that provide meaningful information on the patient's health status and state of balance. Adaptive mechanisms can be identified to indicate balance-seeking behaviors.

4. Cultural data

The use of **cultural data** in the total assessment of the patient cannot be overemphasized. Everyone comes from a cultural background and culture influences behavior, beliefs, relationships, and practices.[2] In the United States, the demographic trend points to an increasingly multicultural population. As the world becomes more inter-connected and globalization has become a reality, people are also becoming more mobile. Populations are also changing in many parts of the world and nurses are finding themselves providing care to a multi-cultural population. It is therefore important for the health care practitioner to understand the cultural data relevant to the client's response to illness and how this can be directed towards balance-seeking behaviors. The concept of balance is specifically identified in many cultures and even perhaps not specifically named, is intuitively present in various aspects of the culture. Relevant cultural data can shed light on people's behavior. Family members and/or significant others present with the patient can give helpful clues about the patient's social and health behaviors.

5. Communication

Related to culture is the patient's ability to **communicate** in the language that is commonly understood between themselves and the health practitioner. It is important to ensure that the patient is able to convey the exact meaning of what he or she is trying to communicate to the health practitioner to avoid misunderstanding. Inability to communicate is a source of frustration between the patient and the provider. If necessary, an interpreter may have to be utilized to facilitate communication. Any source of inability to communicate must also be examined, such as physical or mental disability, and should be considered in the assessment.

6. Maturational/developmental level

One important factor to consider in a health assessment is the **maturational level** of the patient. Chronological age is the objective data related to maturational age. There are different developmental tasks in each age group from infancy to older adult hood and these need to be considered in health assessments. Interview styles and techniques used in assessment also vary with each age group. Young children in particular, especially the chronically ill or disabled, should be approached differently from an adult. In this assessment tool, maturational level is divided into three subgroups: Pediatric (0-18 years), adult (>18-65 years) and older adult (> 65 years). The very young and the very old have risk factors that deserve special consideration. Physical, emotional, and mental status between age groups vary widely and their differences could be significant. Developmental theories should be applied in understanding these differences.

7. Older adults consideration

Although most **older adults** are healthy and living in their community, their lifestyle needs and health issues make them a special concern for nurses. They constitute a large percentage of the population that nurses serve. Some health issues affecting older adults include the following: health promotion, self-management, nutritional awareness, physical fitness and mobility, stress management, accidents, drug use and misuse, mental health/behavioral health problems, and elder neglect or abuse.[1]

8. Functional health patterns

An important source for developing a health assessment tool is the patient's **functional health patterns** to identify positive functions, find dysfunctional health patterns or potential dysfunctional patterns, and identify risk conditions or problems. An assessment tool using the **Gordon's functional health patterns** [1,3] can be used as a framework. Information gathered about the patient can be obtained not just from the patient but also from others who are familiar with the patient's health history and patterns. These include the family, significant others, and other health professionals. In particular, the physician who has taken care of the patient, has made a medical diagnosis, or treated the patient's medical problems, is most familiar with the medical history. However, nurses obtain the most comprehensive data about patients because the assessment tools that nurses use are more geared towards looking at all aspects of the patient—physically, physiologically, psychologically, emotionally, spiritually, and culturally. A health assessment tool with a **holistic approach** that covers all these aspects obtains the most comprehensive database regarding the patient's health status.

COMPONENTS OF THE BALANCE HEALTH ASSESSMENT TOOL

A complete health assessment includes an initial health history and a physical assessment.[11] The assessment tool was designed with several features and components that are specifically geared towards the basic foundation of the Balance Health Nursing Model. The balance model draws its theoretical underpinnings from these various elements: the core elements of balance, theories of behavior and personality, theories of nursing, the internal and external environments, underlying systems and theories of behavior, behavior pyramid, cultural influences, and the health-wellness-illness continuum. These are all explained in the previous chapters of this book. All of these theoretical foundations narrow down to *the basic concept of balance, the basic ingredient of survival.* Without this basic ingredient in the recipe of life, there cannot be life as we know it. And without life, nurses would not find a reason for being. Because nursing is geared towards caring for live patients, restoring their health, maintaining their health, and preventing them from dying become their mandate.

1. Demographic data, general survey, cultural background, and health history

The first part of the tool contains basic demographic information about the patient: name, date of contact, age, maturational level and chief complaints or the reason(s) for the visit. An initial general survey is recorded to document the presenting picture of the patient. The general survey is the provider's statement of their general impression of a patient.[3,11] This includes the initial vital signs measurements, facial expression, body language, position or posture, and signs of pain or discomfort. Pain is considered the fifth vital sign and is one of the first things assessed upon initial contact with the patient. It is a universal, complex, and subjective experience and often an important reason to seek medical attention.[1] Pain alone can alter the patient's physiological, emotional, and mental balance but its presence and severity can be described only by the patient. The location of the pain and its severity on a scale of 0 to 10 (0 is no pain and 10 being the most severe) are part of the initial assessment.

Users of health care services come from all kinds of backgrounds, gender, age, socio-economic status, and culture. These are important considerations in defining who the client is. Developmental stage or maturational level is also an important consideration, not just related to chronological age. It is related to communication and the patient's ability to describe his symptoms and history. There are many factors that contribute to communication issues and this difficulty is initially identified. If the problem is language, then the need for an interpreter could be immediately established before proceeding with the assessment.

Pertinent health history and previous illnesses that contribute to the patient's health status are included. The medications and therapies currently taken are documented, including use of complementary and alternative therapies. It is important to include those because medications and treatments affect patients in many ways. It can be determined if the patient is able to obtain relief of their symptoms from these medications and treatments. Herbal remedies and medications are used by some patients for symptom relief but these may interact with certain medications they are taking. Relevant cultural data such as ethnicity, health and religious beliefs and practices must be included.

Other cultural information that contribute to a better understanding of the patient's health status should be part of the assessment, such as language, food practices, symptom management, illness beliefs, and health promotion activities. All of these information contribute toward increased cultural competencies and culturally appropriate nursing care.[2,5] The presence of family or significant others provides a snapshot of a social aspect of the patient and they can give other relevant information.

2. **Health status indicators: Quantitative and Qualitative data**

The bulk of patient data is contained in the section devoted to **health status indicators** that are both **quantitative** and **qualitative**. Quantitative data are those that are obtained from physiologic assessment of the body systems:[1,7] neurologic/cognitive, respiratory/ventilation, cardiovascular/circulation, renal/urologic, digestive/nutritional, endocrine/hormonal, reproductive function, and musculo-skeletal/ Integumentary. Quantitative data are obtained from accepted standards of measure, such as blood pressure and temperature readings, heart rate, size of a wound, oxygen saturation, fluid intake measurements, number of times patient voids, electrolyte values, blood type, abdominal girth, etc. These data are also obtained through physical examination methods of inspection, auscultation, palpation, and percussion. These physiologic systems assessments are arranged according to their priority of importance to the health status of the patient—**primary assessments** are done first and **secondary assessment** are done next. The systems that are essential to survival are given first priority such as the neurologic, respiratory and cardiovascular systems following the CPR (cardiopulmonary resuscitation) guidelines of the American Heart Association.[8] This guideline is always useful in prioritizing the most vital needs of the patient: (A) air or oxygen, (B) breathing, (C) circulation. Without these critically important functions, the survival of the patient can be immediately jeopardized. The most healthy patient can deteriorate very rapidly without oxygen, if breathing ceases, or circulation collapses. In Maslow's Hierarchy of Needs, these physiologic elements are the most basic for survival.

Secondary assessments follow the primary assessments to determine physiologic functions of those other body systems that are also important for its functioning but not immediately needed, such as fluids or water, nutrition or food intake, hormonal regulation, skin and muscle integrity and reproduction. Underlying all these is the need for safety, the preservation of the physical integrity of the human being, and to be free from danger or risk from death or extinction.

Qualitative or subjective data are those that are reported directly by patients and reflect the patients' own perception of their problems.[9] Examples of subjective data reported by patients are pain, anxiety, feeling guilty, discomfort, mental distress, distrust, depression, sadness, joy, and a whole variety of feelings and emotions that only the patient can describe. The patient's own perceptions and experiences dictate their responses and behavior reflecting these. Behaviors that are inconsistent with what the patient states need to be evaluated further to determine if these data are valid. For example, a patient who reports "severe pain" and yet appears comfortable and sleeping soundly in bed, need to be evaluated. A pain scale of 0 to 10 is used by health care practitioners to quantify the patient's pain level, with 0 as no pain and 10 as the most severe pain. The level reported by the patient is taken at face value but also evaluated for confirmatory evidences such as physiologic signs of pain—sweating, increased heart rate, or increased blood pressure.

The qualitative or subjective data obtained in the Balance Health Assessment Tool also give the nurse an insight into the realm of behavior where the patient appears to be in the Behavior Pyramid—emotional/spiritual, intellectual/rational, or the self-fulfillment stage. The realms of behavior in the Behavior Pyramid and the needs in Maslow Hierarchy are not totally well-delineated and these can overlap each other. For example, safety and security needs and love and belonging needs in Maslow's Hierarchy may fall within the emotional and spiritual realms in the Behavior Pyramid. Self-esteem needs may be part of the intellectual/rational realm in an individual's need for self-fulfillment. Human behavior is so complex that no one theory can explain all its nuances. By knowing these theoretical frameworks of needs and behaviors, the nurse can utilize this knowledge in understanding patients' behaviors and motivations, and thus formulate an individualized nursing care.

3. **Evidences of balance and imbalances: Normal vs. abnormal**

Indicators provide evidences in the determination of whether a certain system or aspect of the patient is in balance or imbalance. **Balance is defined as *within normal limits*** of physiological and psychological behavior as determined by quantitative and qualitative indicators (evidences). **Imbalance** is when the values are outside the range of normal. For instance, a normal state of balance in the neurologic system is for the patient to be awake, alert, and able to respond appropriately to verbal stimuli or commands. The normal or balance column is then checked. If the patient is confused, incoherent, unable to follow verbal commands, this is abnormal and falls within a state of imbalance. Indicators or evidence of this imbalance must be described and documented in a concrete and concise manner on the appropriate space provided on the form. Another example is the respiratory system indicator of breathing pattern. Respiratory rate can be affected by many variables such as age, disease, activity, body temperature.[1,10] Respiratory changes in young children and older adults must be particularly considered. Normal respiratory rate for an adult is 14 to 20 breaths per minute. Normal breathing pattern should be regular, even, and effortless. Breathing that falls outside this range is abnormal and places the patient in a state of imbalance. Again, this finding should be documented on the form under the "imbalance" (abnormal) column.

Physiologic evidences of imbalance are easier to identify because they are measureable and quantifiable. Psychological evidences are more difficult because they are subjective and qualitative. This means that these can only be determined and verified by the patient himself or herself based on their individual perceptions and personal standards. Because experiences and perceptions vary from one individual to another, quantifying these can be extremely difficult. There are no instruments developed at this time to quantify all human emotions based on individual variables. Imbalances can be based on common frames of reference within that particular society, group or culture. Ultimately, it is the patient who decides whether this is an imbalance in their perception or not. For example, a person who is deeply affected by a negative relationship with a family member may be in a state of emotional imbalance if he or she is unable to use normal coping mechanism. The patient may exhibit abnormal behaviors such as suicidal gestures, which place this person in a state of imbalance. Inability to deal with stress such as work or family demands could lead to abnormal behaviors such as alcoholism or aggressive behaviors. These should be documented as abnormal behavior and an evidence of imbalance. It is also important for the nurse to have a background knowledge of psychology and mental health principles to be able to identify psychological problems.

4. **Functional level**

Functional level was included as part of the assessment because it is also important in the determination of the patient's health status. Functional level is an overall assessment of the ability of the patient to be able to function physically, mentally and emotionally to deal with activities of daily living. There are three functional levels:

Level 1 is fully independent—patient is fully independent and able to take care of his/her own needs and activities of daily living without having to rely on others.
Level 2 is partially independent—patient is able to take care of some his/her own needs and activities of daily living part of the time; relies on others to perform some tasks which they cannot perform.
Level 3 is totally dependent—patient is not able to take care of any of his/her own needs and completely relies on others to take care of them, including activities of daily living and basic survival functions like eating, drinking, and elimination. These are patients who are totally incapacitated and unable to perform even the most basic activities of daily living.

5. Remarks are miscellaneous statements that the nurse want to include that are not covered in any of the other categories but feels that the additional information is important in the assessment.

6. Nursing Diagnosis is a statement that describes the patient's response to an imbalance problem based on the assessment data and prioritized according to the patient's needs which can be resolved through nursing interventions. It is a clinical judgment of the patient's behavioral response to an actual or potential imbalance problem evidenced by assessed data and used as basis for definitive nursing interventions. The nursing diagnoses identified then become the basis for writing an individualized nursing care plan which is used by all members of the nursing team.

(See Balance Health Assessment Tool form—Table 10.1)

CASE STUDY: AN APPLICATION OF THE BALANCE HEALTH ASSESSMENT TOOL:

Initial survey and demographic information

Mrs. Cruz, a 70-year old woman from the Philippines, was admitted to the Medical/Surgical unit of a local hospital in the San Francisco Bay area complaining of shortness of breath on exertion, weakness, fever of five days' duration, coughing thick yellow sputum, painful chest when coughing, and poor appetite. She is widowed for 10 years and lives with her married daughter and her three young grandchildren, ages 12 years, 9 years and 5 years. She was a high school teacher in the Philippines and was petitioned by her daughter to come to the United States after her husband died. She takes care of her grandchildren full time while her daughter and son-in-law are at work. She complains of chest pain when she coughs.

Her baby-sitting responsibilities only allowed her to meet other members of the local Filipino community during weekends at church and during occasional social gatherings. Without her husband, she feels quite lonely and often thinks of going back to the Philippines, although she loves her grandchildren dearly. However, her daughter has begged her to stay and help take care of the three grandchildren. She misses her friends and other relatives in the Philippines but torn between her family obligations with her daughter.

She has a history of hypertension which is currently being treated with maintenance oral hypertensives, and borderline diabetes which is not being treated. Like most immigrant Filipinos, she likes to eat native foods like "adobo" (a chicken or pork meat dish with soy sauce and vinegar), "pinakbet" (a vegetable dish with fish sauce), and sweet delicacies. She is also a very religious woman and prays the rosary every night.

According to her daughter, she has not been able to drink and eat adequately for the last three days because of poor appetite and fever. Coughing has kept her awake at night. She took some herbal remedies and liniments, such as a cough syrup from a herbal plant ("lagundi") she had brought from the Philippines to ease her symptoms. She avoids cold drinks and did not shower for three days because she believes that these will make her symptoms worse. She keeps her room closed to avoid draft for fear of "bad wind". She takes multivitamin supplements daily to "keep her strong".

Initial admission survey data revealed an awake but slightly lethargic elderly Filipino female with cheeks flushed lying in a high fowler's position in bed; complaining of cough productive of thick yellow sputum and thirst; appears anxious and weak. She says her chest "hurts" when she coughs, pain level 8 on a scale of 0 to 10. Primary assessment revealed the following: respiratory rate 36/min., slightly labored with some audible wheezing; blood pressure 110/80; heart rate 120/min., weak, and slightly irregular; temperature 102.6 degrees Fahrenheit; skin very warm, and face flushed.

Primary admitting diagnosis: **Pneumonia;** secondary diagnosis: **dehydration, rule/out cardiac disease.** Per admitting orders of the physician, oxygen was immediately initiated at 4 liters per minute via nasal cannula and an IV infusion of Dextrose 5% in 0.45% saline solution at 100 cc. per hour was started on the left forearm. Other orders included: 1) portable chest x-ray ; 2) laboratory tests: arterial blood gases on room air, CBC (complete blood count), electrolyte panel, blood glucose, BUN, creatinine, liver panel, sputum for culture and sensitivity; 3) medications: ceftriaxone sodium one gram IV every 12 hours; acetaminophen (Tylenol) 500 milligrams orally every 6 hrs. for temperature > 101 degrees Fahrenheit; 4) diet: soft diet, encourage fluid intake; 5) measure intake and output; 6) continuous pulse oximetry; 7) 12-lead electrocardiogram, 8) activity: bed rest with bathroom privileges with assistance if tolerated.

Quantitative/objective data: physiologic systems indicators

A. Primary physical Assessment

1. Neurologic/cognitive function

In making the initial assessment of the patient's condition, whether the setting is on a medical-surgical unit, the emergency room, or critical care unit, it is important to follow a certain order of assessment. Basic life support guidelines of the American Heart Association[8] follows definite steps to evaluate the status of the patient to determine if he/or she is in an immediate or potential danger to life and survival. This order should provide a guide to any assessment of a patient in any setting. Prioritization of assessment can spell the difference between life and death. If there are no immediate signs of danger to survival, then the next assessment steps could be performed.

The neurologic function is assessed first to determine the patient's responsiveness and **level of consciousness** (LOC) Neurologic functions are controlled by the nervous system and responsible for monitoring and controlling all aspects of the body's activities within its vast and highly complex network of nerve cells. It is divided into two systems: the central nervous system composed of the brain and spinal cord, and the peripheral nervous system composed of cranial and spinal nerves. Vital centers such as that for breathing, control of heart rate, and blood pressure are contained in the brain stem, as well as that for level of consciousness.

Any change in the level of consciousness or responsiveness gives an indication of the status of brain's vital functions. This is why the primacy of assessing consciousness takes precedence over any other system assessment.

Mrs. Cruz is conscious but lethargic, which indicates that her level of consciousness is not optimum. The reason for this change in her level of consciousness needs to be further assessed. There are several factors that contribute to this condition, including diminished oxygen supply to the brain, metabolic factors, infection, medications, surgery, electrolyte imbalances, and glucose level. Sleep and rest patterns contribute to levels of alertness. Lack of sleep for three days has a depressive effect on neurologic function and could be a factor. However, other conditions may have contributed to it as well.

2. Respiratory/ventilation system

The respiratory system facilitates exchange of oxygen and carbon dioxide between the atmosphere and the blood called **ventilation**. Since oxygen is vital to life, any interference in this process produces immediate consequences to the body. The system requires several components: a patent airway, a supply of oxygen required by the body, ability to move the gases through the respiratory passageway, movement through alveolar-capillary membranes, blood supply to carry oxygen to the cells and ability to remove carbon dioxide. This process happens automatically, regulated by the respiratory center in the brain, whether one is asleep or awake. This vital function is a requirement for human beings to survive. Many factors affect the rate and depth of respirations, such as developmental stage, infections, presence of acute or chronic illness, structural or anatomic defects, medications, neurological conditions, metabolic disorders, cardiac problems, trauma, emotional distress, among others. Respiratory symptoms are often manifestations of problems in other parts of the body.[1,3]

The presence of respiratory efforts should be immediately assessed in a patient upon presentation to the health care provider. Any abnormality should be noted and if necessary, intervention should be initiated right away. In emergency situations, a rescuer can open the airways and blow into the person's mouth to deliver oxygen. If the patient has spontaneous respirations and awake, patient is administered with oxygen as soon as possible to prevent further deterioration of the respiratory status. As respiratory status is closely linked with cardiovascular status, the cardiovascular function should also be assessed almost simultaneously.

The respiratory pattern of Mrs. Cruz suggests a dysfunction because of the faster rate (32/min.) and the character of her breathing which is slightly labored. There are also audible sounds like **wheezing** and **rhonchi** upon examination which suggests some impediment in the airways which could be caused by secretions. Her history suggests respiratory disorder since she admits to have been coughing for the past several days with fever. Oxygen was administered right away as ordered by the physician to alleviate her respiratory difficulty. A monitoring device (pulse oximeter) was attached to her finger to determine her oxygen saturation and pulse rate. Arterial blood gas (ABGs) was ordered—a test using arterial blood to assess acid-bases balance, ventilation status, and need for oxygen therapy.

3. Cardiovascular/circulation

The circulatory system enables oxygen, food materials, and other chemicals to reach every cell of the body to keep it alive. Without those life-giving elements, even the most simple of organisms cannot survive. The circulatory system acts as the transport system, composed of a pumping mechanism (the heart), blood and fluids that carry life-giving elements, and the vessels from the largest to the tiniest for transport of materials to and from the cells. It carries by-products of metabolism, including carbon dioxide, away from the cells to be removed by other systems. Any failure of the pump, blockage in the vessels or tubings, and leakage in the system, would compromise this closed system. The heart is a powerful organ that has muscles that can automatically beat non-stop but also regulated by a specialized nervous tissue called the **sinuatrial node** (SA) that generates electrical impulses that travel through the muscle fibers of the heart, and enables it to contract and pump blood to and from its four **chambers:** right and left atrium and right and left ventricles. Blood from the right side of the heart is pumped to the lungs for oxygenation via the pulmonary artery; blood from the left side of the heart is pumped to the rest of the body via the pulmonary vein into the aorta. The left ventricle is especially equipped with thick muscles to generate the force necessary to overcome higher pressure from the lower extremities and pump blood to the rest of the body. The heart valves keep blood from flowing back against the flow of circulation. The heart itself has its own blood supply called the **coronary circulation.**[1,3]

The cardiovascular/circulatory system is a top priority assessment for obvious reasons. This includes measurement of the blood pressure, heart rate and pulses. Blood pressure is measured traditionally with a sphygmomanometer and stethoscope, or digitally, using more modern digital blood pressure instruments. Heart rate is assessed by listening to the heart using the stethoscope. It can also be measured using a cardiac monitor that displays the electrical pattern of the heart beat or an **EKG** machine to diagnose conduction abnormalities. Pulses reflect the force of the heart beat against the wall of an artery that can be palpated or felt with the fingers or heard through the stethoscope. A weak pulse indicates that the force of the heart contraction is not as strong or the circulating blood volume is not adequate. An irregular pulse indicates a disruption in the normal rhythm of the heart. Weak pulses and irregular pulses can indicate various cardiac or circulatory conditions.

On examination, Mrs. Cruz had a blood pressure of 110/70, but with a weak and irregular pulse. She had no chest pain, which indicates no acute cardiac condition at this time. However, an irregular pulse signals some abnormality of heart rhythm which needs to be assessed right away. **Dysrhythmias** are abnormalities of cardiac rhythm. An accurate interpretation of this finding should be done right away to evaluate its hemodynamic effect on the patient. Some dysrhythmias are benign and some are lethal. Some causes include electrolyte disturbances, fever, decreased cardiac output, hypotension, and hypoxia. Decreased oxygen supply to the cardiac muscle due to a number of causes need immediate intervention by administration of oxygen. A low blood pressure is caused by other factors and not necessarily cardiac in origin. The primary assessments of the neurologic status, respiratory/ventilation system, and cardiovascular/circulation systems are critical indicators that should be assessed within the first few minutes of contact with the patient.

B. **Secondary physical examination**

1. Renal/urologic system

The maintenance of the renal/urologic function is one of the keys to survival. The kidneys affect all the organs of the body and kidney failure could inevitably lead to death of the organism. The primary function of the kidneys is to filter blood and maintain the body's internal physiologic balance or **homeostasis.** Adequate kidney functioning is essential to the maintenance of balance and health. This is the reason for placing kidney assessment as the first in the second tier of the Balance Health Assessment.

Mrs. Cruz' renal function is compromised because of her history of not taking adequate amounts of fluids. One indication is her poor **skin turgor** upon examination. Her urinary output is decreased because of inadequacy of circulating blood volume from decreased fluid intake. This in turn affects the amount of urine output. The process of urine formation is the outcome of multiple steps involving filtration, reabsorption, secretion, and excretion of water, electrolytes, and metabolic waste products.[3] Adequate fluid intake is important to kidney function. Decreased fluid intake leads to dehydration, a major cause for kidney failure, urinary tract infection, and kidney stones. Assessment of voiding pattern gives a clue to the amount of urine the patient is eliminating.

2. Digestive/nutritional

In Maslow's Hierarchy of Needs, food is one of the basic elements for survival. This involves the digestive system responsible for ingestion, processing, and absorption of food to maintain adequate nutrition and provide fuel for the functioning of the cells. **Nutrition** is the process by which the body uses food for energy, growth, and tissue repair. The digestive process starts with eating and dietary practices of the individual. There are numerous factors that influence eating habits, attitudes, and food preferences, including cultural, religious, socio-economic, and personal factors. It is important to assess not just the intrinsic physical capability of the individual to take, digest, and absorb food, but also the extrinsic factors that affect digestion and nutrition. Lack of food or nutrition will result in malnutrition and metabolic imbalances caused by deficiencies of essential food elements. In extreme cases, starvation lead to death if food cannot be accessed.

Mrs. Cruz prefers food that she is most familiar with because of her cultural practices. Her nutritional status is affected by her illness, lack of appetite, and preference for Filipino foods. She has not been eating well for three days and this places her at risk for nutritional imbalance. This in turn affects her ability to fight infections and provide cellular nutrition necessary for overall healthy functioning of her body.

3. Endocrine/hormonal

In coordination with the nervous system, the endocrine system releases chemical substances called **hormones** that play a role in energy regulation, growth, development, and reproduction through various glands in the body.[2] The effects of these hormones on target cells, tissues, and organs of the body make the endocrine system so critical to the survival of human beings. Hormones not only control many physiologic activities but also human behavior. For instance, it plays a part in stress response via the adrenal glands. One of the more common effects of endocrine function is on the pancreas which regulates glucose and insulin production. **Diabetes**, a disease related to abnormality in insulin production, impaired utilization of insulin, or both, is a prevalent health problem especially among older adults.

Aging contributes to the development of late-onset diabetes which Mrs. Cruz is probably developing. The fact that she has borderline diabetes per her admission, indicates that there is an imbalance in her glucose-insulin metabolism. Genetics, age, and ethnicity are factors that contribute to this condition. Quantitative indicators such as fingerstick blood sugar provide a measure of the level of glucose in her blood at a given time. This was ordered by the physician on admission to evaluate this condition and treat it if necessary.

4. Musculoskeletal/Integumentary

Human beings interact with their external environment to access basic elements of survival such as air, water, and food. They are also equipped with sensory apparatus to receive stimuli from the external environment and react to these stimuli to ensure their survival, well-being, and safety. Stimuli received by the integumentary system thru the skin triggers thermo-regulating and protective mechanisms by the body. These capacities are made possible through the musculoskeletal/integumentary system that also protects the human organism's internal organs and systems. The bony structure of the musculoskeletal system provides the supporting framework and prevents it from collapsing. The skin encases the body with an external protective covering. Besides these protective features, the bones also functions in blood cell production and mineral storage. Activity, exercise, and good nutrition maintain the optimum functioning of these bony structures. Injury to the musculoskeletal system disables the individual and/or limits their ability for movement and locomotion—all essential to well-being.

A survey of Mrs. Cruz's musculoskeletal system reveals no active disease but she has risk potentials due to dehydration and lack of activity and exercise. Poor muscle turgor predisposes to skin breakdown exacerbated by immobility and inactivity. These risk factors need to be considered to prevent future skin and bone injuries.

5. Hematological

The hematological system involves the blood and blood-forming tissues such as the bone marrow, blood elements, spleen, and the lymphatic system. The transport of oxygen and carbon dioxide depend on the ability of body element hemoglobin to combine with oxygen for transport via the cardiovascular system to all the cells of the body. Without this ability to provide oxygen and remove carbon dioxide, cells die and eventually cause death of the entire organism. The birthplace of the elements found in the blood is the bone marrow in the central core of the bone. As the cells mature, these are released into the blood stream to perform various functions such as transport of gases, (oxygen and carbon dioxide), coagulation, and protection of the body from infections. The blood's formed elements and plasma are mixed with body water to constitute both intracellular and extracellular fluids. Body water acts as the solvent of body salts, nutrients, and wastes transported throughout the body. It contains important electrolytes, which are electrically charged particles and essential in water movement to and from the cells. Body water and electrolytes play an important role in **homeostasis**—the internal regulation of metabolic body processes that are essential for survival. Blood loss when not replaced depletes circulating blood volume and poses immediate risk to the person's life.

If Mrs. Cruz has decreased capacity to produce **hemoglobin** and has iron deficiency due to poor nutrition, her ability to carry oxygen to her cells is also impaired. This exacerbates the problem of cellular oxygenation which is already compromised from a respiratory system imbalance. Although her hematological system is not severely jeopardized, this state of imbalance, if allowed to persist, can result in a generalized imbalance of the body.

Qualitative/Subjective data

Subjective data or qualitative data are the patient's own description about his or her health problems based on experiences and perceptions. Only the patient can provide this kind of information. They usually include feelings such as anxiety, concerns, discomfort or pain, emotions, or mental stress. These feelings cannot be objectively measured by any standard measuring instrument and therefore, these cannot be easily quantified. Pain, a common subjective complaint, is usually measured on a scale or 0 to 10, with 0 being no pain and 10 the most severe pain. But then again, this is measured according to the patient's self-rating. Neurophysiological changes accompany the stress experience of the patient and this must be part of their assessment and help validate the patient's description of pain symptoms.

Subjective data can also include the patient's description of family relationships and psychosocial issues, such as relationship with others at work. Stress sources are qualitative data because they are highly specific feelings and perceptions unique to the individual person. What is stressful to one person may not be stressful to another. Possible stress sources include economic issues, political issues, environmental factors, sexuality, death of another person, divorce, care giving, job loss, homelessness, moving to a different residence, social isolation, and any psychosocial factors that the person is unable to cope with psychologically. Culture plays a major role in defining what are stressful to the individual and as well as the coping mechanisms used to deal with the stress factors.[12] Their stress response or coping behavior is also culturally defined. Spirituality and religious beliefs are also culturally influenced. Coping strategies in many cultures are strengthened by their religious beliefs. Their religious beliefs serve to keep the individual in an emotional balance which no amount of medical intervention can suffice. Lack of information or knowledge contributes to stress and nurses must include teaching as part of their intervention.

Subjective data on Mrs. Cruz includes her complaint of chest pain when she coughs, feeling of anxiety, and discomfort. She verbally stated that she had not been able to sleep for the past few days, poor appetite and fever. She rates her chest pain on coughing as 8 on a scale of 0 to 10. Some of her subjective complaints can be validated quantitatively such as her fever, cough and poor appetite. Her temperature was elevated (102.6 degrees F), productive coughing can be observed, and poor appetite validated by her weight loss of 10 pounds (she normally weighs 120 pounds, now weighs 110 pounds). Her lethargy may be related to her lack of sleep for several days.

There is a preponderance of cultural data regarding Mrs. Cruz that can give a more detailed picture of her physical and psychological status. To be able to provide culturally competent care, nurses must be able to understand the culture of the client and how it affects their attitudes and behavior. The patient's ethnic background, health practices and beliefs, and

culture-bound behaviors,[6,13] provide insights into her current health status. Culture bound refers to behavior that reflects the person's sense of "reality" within that particular culture, including their illness behavior. Nurses also come from different cultural backgrounds and bring their own cultural perspective into the nurse-patient interaction. They are also culturally bound within the perspective of their profession, which come from the scientific approach. To bring these two different perspectives together in providing culturally appropriate and competent care is a challenge to the nurse. The balance approach in the Balance Health Nursing Model considers the patient's most basic need—the need for balance within their cultural reality. Mrs. Cruz's attitudes and beliefs about the causes of her illness and culturally-influenced psychological factors affecting her have to be understood and considered in the whole assessment.

Functional Level

An overall assessment of the patient's functional level has to be determined with the initial assessment to obtain a general point of reference of the patient's ability to physically perform activities of daily living. Physical independence is the indicator of a full functional level. At the most basic level, she should be able to perform toileting, hygiene, self-feeding, positioning, getting in and out of bed, communicate or use communication devices, and be entirely aware of her surroundings. This functional level may change on a day to day basis depending on the patient's progress. The goal of nursing care is to help bring the patient to a fully independent functional level in preparation for eventual discharge.

Mrs. Cruz is not able to be fully independent at this time of her hospitalization. She is still weak and lethargic and unable to perform basic activities. She requires assistance with personal hygiene and getting in and out of bed to ensure her safety.

Nursing Diagnosis

The next step after obtaining data from the health assessment tool is to formulate nursing diagnoses based on the imbalances identified for use in an individualized nursing care plan. Assessment is the deliberate and systematic process of obtaining data to determine a client's present and past health status, functional status, functional health patterns, and coping patterns.[9,14] The process of analysis and clustering of the data collected results in a diagnosis of the patient's responses to health care problems. The Balance Health Nursing Model's approach is to focus on imbalances in the various systems of the body through physiologic indicators, and psychological imbalances through qualitative indicators, including cultural data, to arrive at nursing diagnoses based on imbalances. The Balance Health Assessment Tool enables the nurse and health practitioners to obtain systematic information with focus on the patient's imbalances and abnormalities that cause the imbalances.

The following are the nursing diagnoses identified, prioritized according Mrs. Cruz's problems and needs:

1. Impaired neurologic response related to disturbance in sleep pattern and/or decreased oxygenation.
2. Ineffective breathing related to decreased airway patency from infection and secretions causing decreased oxygenation.
3. Impairment in cardiac efficiency related to irregular heart beat and inadequate body fluids.
4. Imbalanced body fluids related to inadequate hydration.
5. Anxiety related to hospitalization and lack of understanding of treatments and interventions.

A sample of Mrs. Cruz's Balance Health Assessment Tool is on the attached sheet.

KEY CONCEPTS
• •

1. The purpose of the Balance Health Assessment Tool is to provide an instrument to obtain initial health assessment data on patients upon entry into the health care system. It is a tool based on the Balance Health Nursing Model that emphasizes focus on the state of balance and evidences of imbalances on a given client. The data obtained will then be used to identify nursing diagnoses for use in the development of an individualized nursing care plan.
2. Several factors are taken into consideration in the tool: focus on balance concepts, prioritization of approach in data gathering, organization and clustering of data, cultural data considerations, communication, maturational/developmental level, older adult considerations, and functional health patterns.
3. Components of the Balance Health Assessment tool include both demographic information, as well as quantitative and qualitative indicators. Quantitative data are measurable physiologic indicators; qualitative are those subjective complaints and non-quantifiable measures that are reported by the patient and/or others. Other components include functional level, and nursing diagnoses.
4. Indicators determine whether a particular system is in balance or imbalance. A balanced state in a particular system means there is no evidence of imbalance or abnormality. An imbalance means that there are evidences or indicators that an abnormality exists. These indicators have to be recorded on the assessment tool.
5. An overall picture of these balance vs. balance indicators and demographic data emerges that lead to the identification of the patient's problems. These are the

statements of the nursing diagnoses, prioritized according to degree of importance to survival.

6. A case study was presented to provide an example of how the tool can be used in real life patients. An elderly Filipino patient living in the United States provided an example of how cultural factors can affect patient's health status, beliefs and perceptions. A culturally appropriate and sensitive approach to care should be part of the nursing care plan. Additionally, considerations for older adults should be included in the plan.

CHAPTER 10: THE BALANCE HEALTH ASSESSMENT TOOL AND APPLICATION

REFERENCES

1. Ignatavicius, D.D. & Workman, M.L. 2006. *Medical-Surgical Nursing: Critical Thinking for Collaborative Care* (5th ed.) St. Louis, Missouri. Elsevier Saunders.
2. Spector, R.E. 2009. *Cultural Diversity in Health and Illness* (7th ed.) Upper Saddle River, New Jersey. Pearson Prentice Hall.
3. Lewis, S.L. et al. *2007. Medical-Surgical Nursing: Assessment and Management of Clinical Problems* (7th ed. South Asia edition) St. Louis, Missouri. Mosby.
4. Gordon, M. 2002. *Manual of Nursing Diagnosis* (10th ed.) St. Louis, Missouri. Mosby.
5. Lipson, J.G. & Dibble, S.L. (Eds.) 2005. *Culture and Clinical care.* San Francisco, California. UCSF Nursing Press.
6. Giger, J.N. & Davidhizar, R.E. 1995. *Transcultural Nursing: Assessment and Intervention* (2nd ed.) St. Louis, Missouri. Mosby.
7. Huether, S.E. & McCance, K.L. 2008. *Understanding Pathophysiology* (4th ed.) St. Louis, Missouri. Mosby.
8. American Heart Association. Highlights of the 2010 American Heart Association Guidelines for CPR and ECC. www.heart.org/heartorg/CPR and ECC/guidelines. (retrieved 3/25/2013).
9. Potter, P.A. & Perry, A.G. 2007. *Basic Nursing: Essentials for Practice* (6th ed.). St. Louis, Missouri. Mosby.
10. Christensen, B.L. & Kockrow, E.O. 2006. *Foundations of Nursing* (5th ed.). St. Louis, Missouri. Mosby.
11. Daniels, R. et al.2010. *Nursing Fundamentals: Caring & Clinical Decision Making* (2nd ed.) Clifton Park, NY. Delmar Cengage.
12. Aldwin, C.M. 2000. *Stress, Coping and Development: An Integrative Perspective.* New York. Guilford Press.
13. Potter, P.A. & Perry, A.G. 2005. *Fundamentals of Nursing* (6th ed.) St. Louis, Missouri. Mosby.
14. Carpenito-Moyet, L.J. 2008. *Nursing Diagnosis: Application to Clinical Practice* (12th ed.) Philadelphia. Lippincott Williams & Wilkins.

BALANCE HEALTH ASSESSMENT TOOL (CASE STUDY)

Nursing Unit:___Medical/Surgical   Unit Date: (date of admission)
Client name: ADELINA CRUZ   Marital status: **Widow** MRN#: *******2345

Age: **70 years** Maturational level: (check one) __Ped (0-18yr.),___Adult(>18-65yr)__**X**_Older adult>65y

Chief complaints/Reasons for visit: **Fever and cough for five days, weakness, chest pain on coughing, shortness of breath, poor food and fluid intake.**

Initial general survey: **70 year old Filipino female lying upright in bed, appears lethargic and weak, responds to verbal stimuli, with slight respiratory difficulty, coughing thick yellow sputum, face flushed.**

Vital signs: **BP 110/80, P 120/min, R36/min. T-102.6 F** Pain level: (0-10) **8** /location: **chest pain on coughing Allergies: None**

Communication issues: Yes _____No **X**. Interpreter needed? Yes____ No **X speaks English well**

Pertinent health history and previous illnesses: **hypertension, slightly elevated blood sugar, hyperlipidemia. Taking prescription medications for hypertension and elevated cholesterol.**

Medications and therapies: (prescribed, herbal and supplements): **Lopressor 100 mg. daily for blood pressure, Lipitor 50 mg. daily for elevated cholesterol, herbal cough medication, multivitamins daily, herbal teas taken daily.**

Relevant cultural data: ex: ethnicity, health and religious beliefs and practices : **Filipino ethnicity; believes in use of herbal remedies for symptoms; hot and cold beliefs with food, hygiene, and environment; deeply religious (Roman Catholic); strong family ties; avoids hospitalizations.**

Check appropriate column:

HEALTH STATUS INDICATORS	Balance (Normal)	Imbalance* (Abnormal) *must document	REMARKS, EVIDENCES OF IMBALANCE (i.e. complaints, labs, exams, findings, etc.)
QUANTITATIVE /OBJECTIVE			
PHYSIOLOGIC SYSTEMS ASSESSMENT			
A. PRIMARY ASSESSMENT			
a. Neurologic/Cognitive			
LOC/Sensory		X	Slightly lethargic
Sleep /rest patterns		X	Lacks sleep—unable to sleep for several days
b. Respiratory/Ventilation			
Lung sounds Breathing pattern		X	Bilateral rhonchi and wheezing rapid breathing, slightly labored
Oxygenation		X	Pulse oximetry 85% room air
c. Cardiovascular/Circulation Heart rate/pulse		X	Heart rate rapid, irregular, pulse slightly weak, face flushed.
Circulation/BP		X	Hx hypertension, now low at 110/70.
B. SECONDARY ASSESSMENT			
d. Renal-urinary			
Fluid intake		X	Inadequate—not drinking fluids x 3 days
Voiding pattern		X	Voids small amounts, dark amber urine,
e. Digestive/Nutritional			
Abdominal survey Nutrition—food intake	X	X	Nutritional intake inadequate, poor appetite
Elimination pattern	X		
f. Endocrine/Hormonal General survey	X		
Blood sugar control		X	Hx. slight blood sugar elevation
g. Reproductive functions			

General survey X

	Balance (Normal)	Imbalance	REMARKS
h. Musculoskeletal/Integumentary Activity/exercise		X	Limited mobility due to weakness
Skin and bone condition		X	Poor skin turgor

i. Hematological Blood-related	X		
B. QUALITATIVE/SUBJECTIVE			
Examples: Pain, discomfort, anxiety, anger, fatigue, etc.			
a. Subjective complaints		X	Level 8 on pain scale, chest pain on coughing, inability to sleep, poor appetite, anxious about hospitalization
b. Psychosocial Family relationships		X	Limited social contacts, lives with daughter, takes care of grandchildren but lonely.
Stress sources		X	Care giving of grandchildren, lack of income, anxiety over health and medical condition.
Spirituality needs	X		Derives emotional comfort in prayers
Knowledge/information needs		X	Lack of understanding about effects of hot and cold on body and medical condition.

FUNCTIONAL LEVEL: (Check one) Level 1____Fully independent; Level 2 **X Partially dependent**; Level3:_____Totally dependent Height___**5 ft. 2in** (Ft/In) __**115 lbs.** Weight(lbs/kilos)_____

REMARKS: **Social Services and dietary consult needed before discharge and possible home health services. Pastoral services for spiritual support.**

NURSING DIAGNOSES : FOR USE IN CARE PLAN* Additional nursing diagnoses on back page

1. Impaired neurologic response related to disturbance in sleep pattern and decreased oxygenation.
2. Ineffective breathing related to decreased airway patency from infections and secretions causing limitation in oxygenation.
3. Impairment in cardiac efficiency related to irregular heart beat and inadequate fluid intake.
4. Imbalanced body fluids and nutrition related to inadequate hydration and poor appetite.

5. Anxiety related to hospitalization and lack of understanding of treatments and interventions.
6. Risk for skin breakdown related to poor hydration and limited mobility.

Completed by: (Print) _____, RN

Signature: _____ Date: _____

TABLE 10.1 BALANCE HEALTH ASSESSMENT TOOL FORM

Nursing Unit:_____Date: _____

Client name: _____Marital status_____ MRN#:_____

Age:__Maturational level: (check one)__Ped (0-18yr.),__Adult(>18-65yr)__Older adult>65y

Chief complaints/Reasons for visit:_____

Initial general survey: _____

Vital signs: BP__P__R__T__ Pain level: 0 to 10 (none to extreme)____/location_____

Allergies: _____

Communication issues: Yes_____No_____. Interpreter needed? Yes_____ No_____

Pertinent health history and previous illnesses:_____

_____

Medications and therapies: (prescribed, herbal and supplements)_____

_____

Relevant cultural data: ex: ethnicity, health and religious beliefs and practices _____

_____

_____

Check appropriate column:

HEALTH STATUS INDICATORS	Balance (Normal)	Imbalance* (Abnormal) *must document	REMARKS, EVIDENCES OF IMBALANCE (i.e. complaints, labs, exams, findings, etc.)
QUANTITATIVE /OBJECTIVE			
PHYSIOLOGIC SYSTEMS ASSESSMENT			
B. Primary assessment			
d. Neurologic/Cognitive			
LOC/Sensory			
Sleep /rest patterns			
e. Respiratory/Ventilation			
Lung sounds			
Breathing pattern			
Oxygenation			
f. Cardiovascular/Circulation			
Heart rate/pulse			
Circulation/BP			
B. SECONDARY ASSESSMENT			
d. Renal-urinary			
Fluid intake			
Voiding pattern			
d. Digestive/Nutritional			
Abdominal survey			
Nutrition—food intake			
Elimination pattern			
h. Endocrine/Hormonal			
General survey			
Blood sugar control			
g. Reproductive functions			

General survey

h. Musculoskeletal/Integumentary Activity/exercise			
Skin and bone condition			
j. Hematological Blood-related			
B. QUALITATIVE/SUBJECTIVE			

Examples: Pain, discomfort, anxiety, anger, fatigue, etc.				
c.	**Subjective complaints**			
d.	**Psychosocial**			
	Family relationships			
	Stress sources			
	Spirituality needs			
	Knowledge/information needs			

Functional level: (Check one) Level 1____Fully independent; Level 2____Partially dependent; Level3:____Totally dependent Height____ (Ft/In)____Weight(lbs/kilos)____

REMARKS:

NURSING DIAGNOSES : FOR USE IN CARE PLAN* Additional nursing diagnoses in back page

1. _____
2. _____
3. _____
4. _____

Completed by: (Print) _____, RN

Signature: _____ Date: _____

TABLE 10.2 EXAMPLES OF NURSING DIAGNOSES BASED ON THE BHNM

Suggested descriptive terms: Imbalanced, impaired, decreased, increased, poor, unstable, unequal, ineffective, intolerance, deficient, risky, inappropriate, acute, diminished, severe, heightened, etc.

	IMBALANCE	NURSING DIAGNOSIS	MANIFESTATIONS: Physiologic and psychosocial indicators
1.	Neurologic (Depressed level of consciousness)	Impaired neurologic response related to decreased cerebral tissue perfusion.	Unresponsive to verbal stimuli, withdraws only to deep painful stimuli, poor gagging reflex, sluggish papillary response to light.
2.	Respiratory (respiratory difficulty)	Ineffective breathing related to diminished airway patency and poor oxygenation.	Rapid respiratory rate >36/min, audible expiratory wheezing, use of accessory muscles of respirations, O2 saturation 85 mmHg., patient states "I have a hard time breathing", sitting upright in bed.
3.	Cardiovascular (cardiac failure)	Diminished tolerance to activity related to impaired cardiac function.	Short of breath on exertion, increased heart rate with activity, inability to perform normal toileting due to fatigue.
4.	Body system fluids (dehydration)	Imbalanced body fluids related to inadequate hydration.	Poor fluid intake, poor skin turgor, dry lips and mucous membranes, low blood pressure, increased heart rate; labs abnormal, malaise.
5.	Musculo-skeletal (leg fracture)	Impaired balance and mobility related to leg pain and bone injury.	Pain on ambulation, unable to maintain balance without crutches, poor tolerance to out of bed activities.
6.	Nutritional status	Imbalanced nutrition related to lack of appetite and poor nutritional intake.	Poor appetite, dislike or intolerance to certain foods, poor caloric intake, weight loss per daily weights.
7.	Sensory (post operative)	Acute pain related to incision from abdominal surgery.	Complained of severe pain 10 out of 10 on pain scale; grimacing and holding on to abdominal area, increased heart rate, diaphoretic.
8.	Psychological state	Depression and anxiety related to concern over breast cancer diagnosis and cultural bias about cancer.	Crying and withdrawn, poor appetite, refuses visitors, insomnia, refuses to have breast examined due to embarrassment and stigma about cancer in culture.
9.	Intellectual	Lack of knowledge regarding new medical diagnosis of diabetes and breast cancer.	Does not understand pathophysiology of the disease, lacks understanding of need for insulin and diet control.
10.	Psychosocial	Withdrawal and depression related to conflict in family relationships.	Refuses to see or speak with family, resentment over daughter's inter-racial marriage and divorce.

THE BALANCE CONCEPT IN HEALTH AND NURSING

Afterword

CHALLEGES FOR THE FUTURE

CHANGING PERSPECTIVES

The world is changing and this fact is part of our daily lives. As the philosopher Heraclitus said five centuries before the birth of Christianity, "Nothing endures but change". The world of the ancients was different from that of the Medieval times; the world we live in at the moment is certainly different from even half a century ago. Perspectives and attitudes also change over time as human beings are constantly buffeted with influences from their external environment. Even the way people communicate is different. Social media has revolutionized the manner by which people connect with each other. The internet is still a brand new world to many, but certainly not to the next generation who will be born with computers as a way of life. Already it is, as I watch my young grandchildren play and navigate on their ipads with ease. I gaze with a sense of wonder at these children who will be living in the world of tomorrow, a world that is now becoming difficult for me to imagine. What would the ancients have thought if they only knew what their world will eventually become?

History tells us that attitudes and practices about health have changed over time, as new discoveries in technology and scientific thought shape our thinking. Health care practices have undergone change as it has with the nursing profession. I remember the time four decades ago when nurses wore nursing caps as a proud symbol of their profession in the United States. While wearing a cap is still practiced in other countries, in the United States the cap has gone the way of an old pair of shoes—discarded and forgotten. So does the white uniform. That crisp starched white uniform still evokes a sense of respect and professionalism for me when I see a nurse wearing a white uniform. It is part of the trappings and traditions of the nursing profession that for some of the older generation of nurses are still hard to let go.

But the perceptions and expectations have changed over the last two decades when nursing means more than just a cap and a white uniform. For the new generation of nurses, it is their knowledge, skills and attitudes that set them apart from the other professions. It is what we take with us to the bedside when we interact with our clients. It is not just what we have contained inside our highly trained and developed brain, but how we perform those actions that define our profession. It is in that indefinable character and behavior borne out of education, knowledge, skills, and an in-depth understanding of the nature and humanity of the clients we serve, that become our badge when we call ourselves a NURSE. Nurses are also dealing with increasingly multi-cultural and multi-generational clients with needs that could be so different from one another. This appears to be a daunting task for all nurses in the profession. Are there commonalities that we can use as a framework in our practice which can make it easier to provide the best care we can possibly give without painting everyone with one broad brush?

As humans ascend the Behavioral Pyramid beyond the physiologic level, more psychosocial needs arise. Other psychosocial needs determine behavior, and it becomes more and more distinctive of behavior that are purely human. This is where the deviation from ordinary animals take place—in the use of its larger and more sophisticated brain to manipulate the external environment in response to innate psychosocial needs. Beyond the need for physiologic elements, physical safety and love, there are needs that we humans seek to fulfill— spiritual, intellectual, and finally, the need for a self-fulfillment in all aspects of our human existence. Balance-seeking behaviors will instinctively direct us towards that need for balance. The penultimate level where humans experience the most level of balance is self-fulfillment, or the "Self-Actualization" level of Maslow's hierarchy. Balance-seeking behaviors are, in a way, our means to ensure our survival. In the process, we find individual satisfactions along that way, like cookie crumbs in life's journey, directing humans to live in the best way possible and finding balance in its path.

My journey of discovery into the meanings of balance and how critical this element is in human survival has led me to believe that balance is a key concept in ensuring the health of nursing clients. In the previous chapters, I have explored the core elements of balance, its related concepts, the internal factors that also determine the manner we respond to stimuli, the influence of culture, the mind-body connection, etc. among others—factors that constitute human survival. What remains as a task in this book is to explore further the cross-cultural application of the Balance Health Nursing Model and how this can help in addressing health care disparities that are still prevalent in U.S. health care systems. Additionally, the rapidly expanding elderly population deserves much closer attention in our health care models. The needs of the elderly are quite different from other groups in the general population. A narrower focus is that of the ethnic elderly, a group that is at greater risk for ill-health but almost invisible within the health care system.

CROSS-CULTURAL APPLICATION

Cesario states that every aspect in one's life (including attitudes, beliefs, and values) is influenced by one's culture.[1] It is now recognized by nursing that providing culturally relevant care is essential to the care of all clients. Culture is an organizing frame of reference when looking at people's behavior. Many theorists of human behavior believe that it is culturally determined and each individual is culturally unique. But culture is dynamic and changes over time as people adapt to their life experiences. It is adaptive in the sense that their values and beliefs are shaped by forces that affect them in their constantly changing external environment. In order for groups to survive and thrive in their environments, they have to summon their natural adaptive capacities as they gain new information and insights into their life circumstances. But because individual or groups experiences vary, these may have given rise to vast cultural differences over time. The diversity of culture appears to be consistent with the diversification of all life forms on this planet. Predictably, diversity in cultures will continue in its trajectory as long as life is propagated far into the future.

The BHNM is predicated on man's ability to respond to internal and external stimuli through balance-seeking behaviors as long as the elements of balance are sustained. Behavioral responses, as we have learned, are culturally determined. Even the innate responses to physiological demands of the body can be altered or pre-determined by cultural practices. The need for food, a basic physiologic need, is met in various ways in different cultures. Food preferences are culturally determined and what are accepted dietary practices in one culture may not be acceptable in others. Balance is a basic concept in the food practices of some cultures. For instance, hot and cold foods (yin and yang principle) in some Asian cultures are balanced in order to prevent illness. For some, food practices are dictated by religious beliefs. In the Muslim religion, *halal* foods are those permitted by Allah, the Supreme Law Giver. Other foods called the *haram*, mostly from animals, are strictly prohibited.[2]

Likewise, spiritual or religious practices differ from one culture to another. The spiritual realm is an area in the Behavioral Pyramid that is a stage of psychosocial development. The origin of this largely unexplored area of human behavior is a fascinating subject left for future discoverers of knowledge. Spirituality is derived from the Latin word *spiritus*, meaning breath or wind.[3] It is believed that the spirit is at the center of all aspects of one's existence and gives life to a person. This belief helps individuals find balance to maintain health and well-being through relationship with a higher power or God, nature, or other people. A person's health, as discussed in the Balance Health Nursing Model is influenced by, and depends on, the balance of physical, psychological, sociological, cultural, developmental, and spiritual factors. Religion, as an expression of spirituality, is an important element of culture that influences behavior in a group of people. Religious rituals, such as caring for the dead and the sick, birth and labor practices, baptism, and worship for a higher power, are practiced in various ways by religions and groups of people such as Christianity, Hinduism, Buddhism, Islam, Shinto, Judaism, and Navajos.[3,4] Spirituality and spiritual well-being are important factors in healing and dealing with stress and major life events. They are important elements in achieving physical and emotional balance. The client's spirituality and religion are important frames of reference in providing caring interventions by nurses and other health care professionals.

The role of culture is especially important for health professionals because of culture's influence on health beliefs, attitudes and practices. As defined by Giger and Davidhizar, "Culture is a patterned behavioral response that develops over time as a result of imprinting the mind through social and religious structures and intellectual and artistic manifestations".[5] Key to understanding of the concept of culture is the idea that culture is part of the totality of human behavior, that one cannot view a person as separate from the milieu of the culture where that person belongs, or identifies with. One's attitudes, beliefs and practices about health, illness, and healing are embedded in a culture. These are changed by many sociological, psychological, environmental, or political influences. Education plays a major role in changing perspectives, attitudes and behaviors. For instance, an Asian-American nurse trained in the United States would have a different view of health and illness from her/ his parents' traditional view. Education has apparently changed the nurse' perspectives. The United States, considered a melting pot of cultures, is seeing an increasing **diversity** of cultures never before seen in its history. This diversity is a crucial element to be considered in caring for multicultural patients in the United States and all over the world.

Cross-cultural competence and sensitivity need to become a more central element to caring in nursing. We have learned in the chapter on culture that the concept of balance is embedded in the cultural beliefs of many people around the world. Culture, as part of the universality of the balance phenomenon serves as a platform for caring for patients regardless of color, ethnicity, religion, language, or socio-economic background. A cultural frame of reference needs to guide approach to nursing and health care practices, more so than ever before. It has to be generated from the individual client's values, meanings, and life patterns that are **culturally congruent**. This concept of culturally congruent care was espoused by Madeleine Leininger as the goal of **transcultural nursing**.[3,6,7] Care that is culturally congruent is that which is compatible with, and generated from, people's own life patterns and meanings. This approach may be different from the values of the professional health care system based on the Western medicine model.

The **holistic** nature of nursing requires an individualized approach that is unique to each client. **Diversity** of cultures and differences of cultural practices even among the same **ethnicity** makes the task of individualized approach a very challenging one. Population census projections show an even more increasing diversity among the minority populations outpacing the majority white populations. Hispanic/Latinos, Asian-Americans, and African Americans are growing faster than the majority whites.[7,8] Diversity in race is accompanied by diversity in languages that is quite mind-boggling. It is not hard to imagine that this could lead to another "Tower of Babel" in the Bible, where there were numerous languages spoken by the people in that place at that time. Since communication is an important component in the nurse-patient interaction, this impacts the nursing process. Ability to understand what the patient is communicating is crucial to identification of problems and arriving at a nursing diagnosis to carry out a nursing care plan. And, as health beliefs, attitudes and practices vary from one culture to another, the task of the nurse to provide culturally congruent and appropriate care becomes a tremendous endeavor. Herein lie the challenges for future nurses providing care in a multicultural world.

ADDRESSING HEALTH CARE DISPARITIES

Access to health care has long been a concern of governments all over the world. The nurse, as part of the health care system, has a stake in this concern because it is nurses' professional obligation to ensure the health of his/her clients. The nurse may think that she is far removed from these concerns because her practice only involves a very tiny fragment of this global population. But the care of one client at a time impacts the larger community, and eventually the nation. Globalization has spread the influence of nurses all over the world and nursing perspectives in health has impacted the way care is delivered. Inability of people to access health care produces disparities that have long-lasting effects from generation to generation. What impacts people now can change their worldview and translates into behaviors and attitudes. A population whose health has not been addressed will continue with the same types of behavior and habits that lead to imbalances in their health and well-being. The human cost of these disparities is hard to imagine and quantify.

Health disparities are essentially those differences in health measures between different groups of people living in a community, a state, or an entire country.[9] The National Institutes of Health in the U.S. defines *health disparities* as differences in the incidence, prevalence, mortality, and burden of diseases and other adverse health conditions that exist among specific population groups in the United States.[10] In the 2011 National Healthcare Disparities Report, it emphasizes this goal of government: "The U.S. health care system seeks to prevent, diagnose, and treat diseases and to improve the physical and mental well-being of all Americans."[11] Furthermore, the report says that it focuses on prevailing disparities in health care delivery as it relates to racial factors and socioeconomic factors in minority populations.

This brings to focus the plight of cultural minority populations who have benefitted less from a modern health care system such as the United States. The factors that contribute to health disparities are: race; culture and ethnicity; geographic location; income; education; occupation; health literacy; gender; age; and health care provider attitudes.[9] The impact of health disparities on health outcomes become more obvious among racial and ethnic minorities in the areas of obesity, chronic illness, hypertension, chronic obstructive pulmonary disease (COPD), cancer and stroke. Furthermore, it was also found out that communication is a big issue in accessing health care among cultural minorities who speak a different language than their providers. Nursing, being the biggest group of health care professionals, is implicated in this finding. Factors such as stereotyping and prejudice can affect health care-seeking behavior in minority populations, according to one study.[12]

The Office of Minority Health under the U.S. Department of Health and Human Services have published (2007) the standards for the National Culturally and Linguistically Appropriate Services (CLAS) in Health and Health Care intended to advance health equity, improve quality and eliminate health disparities with this principal standard: "Provide effective, equitable, understandable and respectful quality care and services that are responsive to diverse cultural health beliefs and practices, preferred languages, health literacy and other communication needs".[13] The unifying element in the goals of government to eliminate health disparities is the importance of culture in the health of its populations. Realizing the increasing cultural diversity that characterizes the United States population, the focus on culturally and linguistically appropriate services is intensified. However, it must be remembered that individuals that belong in each culture are also individually unique— each one bringing a perspective entirely one's own. Each person is a product of the internal and external forces that shaped the human race. And yet, herein is a dichotomy: while each individual is different, each one also shares the commonality of balance. In the end, this is the element that binds us all. Eliminating health disparities starting with culturally appropriate individualized care balances that equation and bridges the health care gap. Incorporating culturally sensitive and congruent care into nursing practices helps restore health and balance into people's lives.

SPECIAL FOCUS ON OLDER ADULTS

The elderly population has seen a phenomenal growth towards the end of the twentieth century and continues to grow into the next millennium. Older adults over 65 years fall into this category. It was reported by the Census Bureau that in July, 2004, 12 percent of all Americans, or 26.3 million, were 65 and over.[14] However, it is projected that people 65 and over will comprise 21 percent of the U.S. population, or 86.7 million, by year 2050. More impressive is the rate of growth of this segment of the population. The projected increase in the 65-and-over population between year 2000 and 2050 is a whopping 147%. Compare that with the percentage increase of only 49 percent of the population as a whole in the same period. The two factors identified as major contributors to this growth are: one, the increase in the number of adults that are aging from the "baby boomers" (adults born between 1946 and 1964), and two, increasing number of the elderly over 85, sometimes called the frail elderly. Better health care, improved nutrition, healthier lifestyles, higher education, and advanced technology all contribute to a longer lifespan and improved quality of life for older people and the general population as a whole.

Older adults have special issues that are different from other age groups. The physical, physiological, cognitive, and psychosocial changes associated with aging are specially challenging to health care professionals. Although an increasing number of older adults are now living healthier and more productive lives, another segment of this population still require different approaches to maximize their potentials and live the rest of their lives in relative productivity as members of society. Nursing assessments must take in consideration some key points related to aging such as: 1) physical and physiologic changes, 2) cognition and memory changes, 3) slower reflexes and decreased physical ability, 4) effects of disease and disability on health, 5) alteration in psychosocial behavior, 6) sleep and sensory disturbance, and 7) pharmacological response to medications. All of these have implications on nursing diagnosis and interventions.

The minority older adult population is one that also deserves attention as their numbers grow increasingly, per U.S. Census Bureau projections.[14] The minority population is composed of African Americans, Hispanics, American Indians/Eskimos/Aleuts, and Asian/Pacific Islanders. Overall, the minorities, currently comprising 37% of the population, are projected to comprise 57 percent of the population in 2060, bringing with it an older population growing at varying rates—the Hispanics increasing dramatically, followed by the Asian/ Pacific, the American Indians/Eskimos, and the African-Americans.[3] The minority older adults, also known as the **ethnic elderly,** have special needs related to their age and culture. Many have immigrated to this country and have different historical experiences from each other. They bring with them many traditional beliefs about health and illness that would challenge the American health care professionals. Nurses must represent the clients from populations they serve. And with the increasing diversity and numbers of the older adults, as well as the ethnic elderly, the task of nurses becomes much more challenging. Minority nurses are needed more than ever to better serve their client population.

Minority nurses also bring their cultural perspectives to the nurse-patient interaction in the nursing process. Unless totally acculturated in the Western culture, their belief systems are probably still be rooted in their unique culture. While they bring their own cultural uniqueness into the nurse-patient interactions, they must also consider the cultural, ethnic, and racial diversity of their clients, as well as the special needs of the ethnic elderly. They have to guide and be a resource to other nurses from other cultures in understanding the ethnic client. Culturally sensitive approaches to the ethnic elderly include food preferences, health and illness beliefs and practices, religious practices, symptom management using herbal remedies, family relationships, birth and death practices, and communication patterns. Ultimately, it is when nurses possess that caring and sensitive attitude towards their clients, putting the client's individual needs foremost, becoming their advocate, and helping them reach balance in their lives through balance-seeking behaviors will they help clients find that zone of equilibrium where optimal health could be achieved—one client at a time. By using the Balance Health Nursing Model, they can provide care that is more cognizant of their client's culture, while practicing with a more universal perspective of upon which the model is based.

BALANCE: A UNIVERSAL LAW OF NATURE?

Laws of nature follow logical patterns and universal applicability. One such set of laws were those formulated by Isaac Newton in the late seventeenth century: 1) the law of inertia, 2) objects in motion, and 3) action and reaction. These are the foundations of his "universal law of gravitation".[15] Although scientists in the twentieth century, such as Albert Einstein, later found that Newtonian laws do not apply in all situations, Newton's laws are still as useful today as when these were formulated over three centuries ago. Many laws have been subsequently formulated by modern scientists and their applicability in modern times are numerous. Without the evolution of scientific thought, these laws would not have come to fruition.

I came across a piece about the late author Richard Wetherill, who identified a natural law of behavior.[16] He and a group of his former students had been presenting this idea for several decades. Noting the escalation of today's problems in society—crime, corruption, wars, mental disorders—he proposed a solution found in creation's natural law of "absolute right". In order to survive, civilization must conform to the creator's formula for life: behavior that is deemed rational and honest. Furthermore, it proposes that when people keep their balance, they are acting on the intent of a natural law. Many natural laws, such as the law of gravitation, govern man's existence.

I see a truism in his philosophy that applies to my own concept of balance. If we consider natural laws discovered by and formulated by man, the concept of balance appears to be part of a constellation of laws in the universe. It is embedded in physical laws, social science laws, economic laws, engineering concepts, and many other fields. It is an indefinable force, energy, need, urge, or striving directing humans towards a zone of balance where the ultimate of survival is found. Could this be a "natural law" that nature intended, and part of human existence the day human life existed? Was this built-in mechanism the law that governs life?

And does human behavior direct us towards this zone—a zone of absolute right to preserve human existence? Perhaps somewhere along the way, humans deviated from this path and resulted in imbalances. I cannot resist this tantalizing thought.

As with any novel idea, I will undoubtedly find critics for its logic, universality, and applicability. But what I know is this: that balance exists in our lives, with or without our control. How we direct our behavior so we could find this ultimate zone is entirely up to us, to our family, community, and others we call our clients. Perhaps, with the help of caring and helping professionals, humans will continue to survive well into the future.

AFTERWORD: CHALLENGES FOR THE FUTURE

REFERENCES

1. Cesario, S.K. 2010. "Culture and Ethnicity". in Daniels, R., Grendell, R.N. and Wilkins, F.R. *Nursing Fundamentals: Caring and Clinical Decision Making (2ⁿᵈ ed.)* Clifton Park, NY. Delmar, p. 98.
2. Lipson, J.G. and Askaryar, R. 2005. "Afghans". In Lipson, J.G. and Dibble, S.L. (Eds.). *Culture and Clinical Care.* San Francisco, CA. UCSF Nursing Press, p. 5-6.
3. Potter, P.A. and Perry, A.G. 2005. *Fundamentals of Nursing* (6ᵗʰ ed.) St. Louis, MO. Mosby.
4. Daniels, R., Grendell, R.N., Wilkins, F.R. 2004. *Nursing Fundamentals: Caring and Clinical Decision Making* (2ⁿᵈ ed.) New York. Delmar Thomson Learning.
5. Giger, J.N. and Davidhizar, R.E. 1995. *Transcultural Nursing: Assessment and Intervention* (2ⁿᵈ ed.) St. Louis, Missouri. Mosby-Year Book, Inc., p. 3.
6. Leininger, M.M. 2002. "Culture Care Theory: a major contribution to advance transcultural nursing knowledge and practices". in *Journal of Transcultural Nursing*, 13(3):189.
7. Byrne, M.M. 2006. "Cultural Aspects of Health". in Ignatavicius, D.D. and Workman, M.L. *Medical-Surgical Nursing: Critical Thinking for Collaborative Care* (5ᵗʰ ed.) St. Louis, Missouri. Elsevier Inc.
8. U.S. Department of Commerce Bureau of Census. 2001. *Population profile of the United States.* Washington, DC: U.S. Department of Commerce. www.census.com. Retrieved 2013.
9. Berkowitz, B. and Heitkemper, M.M. 2007. "Health Disparities". in Lewis, S.L. et al. *Medical Surgical Nursing: Assessment and Management of Clinical Problems* (7ᵗʰ ed.). St. Louis, Missouri. Mosby.
10. First National Institutes of Health Work Group on Health Disparities. http://healthdisparities.nih.gov/whatare.html. accessed March, 2013.
11. Highlights from the 2011 National Healthcare Quality and Disparities Reports. http://www.ahrq.gov/research/findingsnhqrdr11/key.html. accessed 4/22/2013.
12. Rathore, S.S., Krumholz, H.M. 2004. "Differences, Disparities, and Biases: Clarifying Variations in Health Care Use". *Ann Intern Med.* 19: 635.
13. National Standards on Culturally and Linguistically Appropriate Services. http://minorityhealth.hhs.gov/templates/browse.aspx. retrieved 4/25/2013.
13. Census Offers Statistics on Older Americans. About.Com US Government Info. http://usgovinfo.about.com/od/censusand statistics/a/olderstats.html. retrieved 4/26/2013.

14. Kauffmann III, W.J. and Freedman, R.A. 1999. *Universe* (5ᵗʰ ed.) New York. W.H. Freeman and Company.

15. The Alpha Publishing House. Intent. http://www.alphapub.com/intent_essay.html. retrieved 5/2/2013.

SELECTED KEY TERMS RELATED TO THE BALANCE, HEALTH, AND NURSING CONCEPTS

The following terms have been selected and defined as used within the context of this book.

Adaptation—The process by which all living creatures on earth modify themselves through many generations to take advantage of their environment and in so doing ensure their survival.

Allopathic—Health beliefs and practices derived from current Western scientific models and uses technology and other modalities to treat diseases and other health conditions in modern health care.

Axis of health—An imaginary vertical line in the health-illness continuum that intersects balance and imbalance centered along the zone of equilibrium. The axis is the where health status may change from balance to imbalance or vice versa. The further away the person moves along the axis from a balance state or health within the zone of equilibrium, the closer to a state of imbalance or illness.

Balance—The dynamic interplay of opposing forces that equalize each other within the internal and external environments of a person. A state of stability achieved when the elements of balance are present as defined by each individual and behaviorally demonstrated.

Balance—seeking behavior—Actions performed by an individual to enable him to survive and thrive by finding fulfillment of his physical, physiologic, mental and psychosocial needs.

Basic need—Something that is necessary for survival of the human being, usually physiologic, such as air, water, nutrition, and elimination.

Behavior—An observable, measurable and describable response to stimuli in the internal and external environments of a person. Behavioral responses are in three realms: 1) physical, 2) physiologic, and psychosocial.

Behavior Pyramid—A conceptual model of behavior based on Maslow's Hierarchy of Needs with ascending realms of behavior to seek balance, from the most basic to the ultimate level of balance. The four realms of behavior are: reflexive or automatic, emotional/spiritual, intellectual/rational, and self-fulfillment. Various factors affect behavior at each level.

Concept—An abstract idea or thought that can be translated into concrete form.

Continuum—A continuous whole, quantity, or series of values or elements.

Coping mechanisms—Are those mechanism used by an individual, consciously or subconsciously, in response to stress to maintain emotional equilibrium.

Culture—A set of values, meaning, practices, beliefs, attitudes, and customs shared by a group of people and passed from one generation to the next.

Disease—A specific illness, disorder, or dysfunction with specific signs and symptoms which cause imbalance and disturbance in the person's health and well-being.

Environments—Are conditions or forces present both within (internal or intrinsic) and outside (external or extrinsic) the person's physical body that directly or indirectly affect the person's behaviors or state of being. Environments are composed of physical, physiological, and psychosocial factors.

Equality—A state of balance where one side is of the same value as the other side; two sides that are equidistant from each other.

Equilibrium—A state of stability or condition wherein influencing and/or opposing forces cancel one another.

Evolution—A gradual and continuous process of development or change from an earlier or original form to its present state or form. Adaptive processes influence evolutionary changes.

Harmony—A quality of balance used to signify a blending of elements that are sensed as pleasing to the individual.

Health—A dynamic state of physical, mental, and social well-being and absence of disease that cause imbalance, and represents a person's effective response to stress from the internal and external environments. It is exhibited as balance-seeking behavior.

Holistic—Dealing with the entire system rather than individual parts. A view or approach that considers all aspects of the person—physical, emotional, mental, spiritual, cultural, social and psychological.

Homeopathic—Health beliefs and practices derived from traditional cultural practices to maintain health, restore health and prevent changes in health status.

Homeostasis—The tendency of an organism or cell to regulate its internal conditions, such as the chemical composition of its body fluids, so as to maintain health and functioning, regardless of outside conditions. The organism or cell maintains homeostasis by monitoring its internal conditions and responding appropriately when these conditions deviate from their optimal state.

Human open system—An open system in human beings possessing permeable boundaries that permit the transmission of physical and psychosocial stimuli and information

Illness—A state of imbalance within the person in relation with the internal and external environment defined and exhibited in the physical, mental, emotional, and psychosocial behaviors of the individual.

Imbalance—A disturbance in balance resulting in a state of relative disequilibrium or instability due to the outweighing of a factor or set of factors over other influencing factors. It is a state when the elements of balance are incomplete and behaviorally demonstrated.

Inputs—stimuli from the internal and external environments in a system that are capable of eliciting a behavioral response from the organism or individual.

Metaparadigm—the most abstract level of knowledge and encompasses the major concepts that provide structure within a discipline. The metaparadigm of nursing are person, environment, health, and nursing.

Model—A theoretical representation of relationships between concepts to understand complex ideas. Nursing models are those models derived from the concepts within the discipline of nursing and also drawn from other disciplines.

Need—Something lacking or deficient that is required or desired by the individual in order to meet a deficiency and produce a state of satisfaction, stability, and equilibrium.

Nursing process—A framework for providing professional nursing care that utilizes systematic problem-solving and critical thinking involving the steps of assessment, nursing diagnosis, planning and outcome identification, implementation, and evaluation.

Objective data—Data that are measureable and observable, obtained from standard measurement instruments, assessment techniques, and diagnostic tests.

Open system—A system that interfaces and interacts with its environments by receiving inputs from and delivering outputs to the outside.

Outputs—Behavior produced from processing of stimuli by the individual within a system.

Personality—Behavioral patterns and physical, personal, and inherited characteristics developed by a person, both consciously and subconsciously, that identifies the uniqueness of a person.

Self-fulfillment—The highest level in the Behavior Pyramid where a complete sense of balance is achieved as defined by the individual, characterized by wholeness, health, well-being, harmony, integration, symmetry, recognition, and respect in a social position in society.

Stability—A steady state of balance where the forces impinging on each other are not exerting energy toward or away from the center of gravity.

Stress—Any force, element, or stimuli that are physical, physiological, or psychological in nature that disturbs a person's state of physical, psychological and physiological balance.

Subjective data—Data from the client's own account, includes feelings, perceptions, and beliefs.

Survival—The ability of a living organism or individual to maintain life or remain alive

Symmetry—A physical beauty of form resulting from balance of design, structure, anatomy, and other characteristics that are found pleasing to the senses.

Synergy—To work together; combined or cooperative action or force.

System—A set of connected or interrelated parts forming a complex whole.

Well-being—A state or feeling of existence characterized by happiness, prosperity, contentment, and health as defined by the individual.

Zone of equilibrium—the area within the health status of an individual where optimal physical, mental, and psychosocial health, balance and equilibrium are achieved within the health-illness continuum.

REFERENCES

Agnes, M. (Ed.) 2002. *Webster's New Dictionary and Thesaurus*. Cleveland, Ohio. Wiley Publishing, Inc.

Daniels, R., Grendell, R.N. & Wilkins, F.R. 2010. *Nursing Fundamentals: Caring & Clinical Decision Making (2nd ed)*. Clifton Park. New York: Delmar Cengage.

Mosby's Dictionary of Medicine, Nursing & Health Professions (7th ed). 2006. St. Louis, Missouri. Mosby Elsevier.

Spector, R.E. 2009. *Cultural Diversity in Health and Illness (7th ed.)* Upper Saddle River, New Jersey. Pearson Prentice Hall.

Venes, D. (Ed.) 2005. *Taber's Cyclopedic Medical Dictionary (20th ed.)*. Philadelphia, PA. F.A. Davis Company.

ABOUT THE AUTHOR

Daisy Magalit Rodriguez practiced as a registered nurse in California where she has resided with her family after immigrating from the Philippines in 1972. She obtained a Diploma in Nursing from the University of the Philippines—Phil. General Hospital School of Nursing; a Bachelor of Nursing and Master in Nursing majoring in nursing administration from the University of the Philippines prior to moving permanently to the United States. She later obtained a second master degree from the University of San Francisco majoring in Public Administration/Health Services. She worked in several acute hospitals in the San Francisco Bay in various capacities from floor nurse to critical care nurse for five years, and later held nursing supervisory positions for over 20 years. She became actively involved in leadership roles in both the local chapter as president, and in the executive board of the national organization of Philippine nurses (PNAA). In 2011, she was named the "Educator of the Year" by PNAA. Her involvement in the community earned her a distinction as one of the "100 Most Influential Filipina Women in the U.S." in 2009 awarded by the Filipina Women's Network. She had a three-year stint teaching in the Philippines and the U.S. prior to her hospital jobs. The last five years of her nursing career was in teaching at an LVN to RN Associate program at Unitek College in Fremont, later becoming the assistant director prior to her retirement in 2012. Her published works include co-authorships in two research projects and two book chapters, as well as having been featured in various articles in the California NurseWeek and Minority Nurse Magazine. Her retirement has allowed her to spend more time reading, ocassionally writing poetry, travelling, and gardening.

Printed in the United States
By Bookmasters